DISC SHMISC

3rd edition

a more accurate model of back pain

Brian Bronk DC

Brian Bronk DC

1821 Wilshire Blvd. #570

Santa Monica, CA 90403

LAbackandbody.com

ISBN 1440454264

EAN-13 9781440454264

Dedication

This book is dedicated to those who suffer in pain.

Who have lost their normal everyday life.

Who have had multiple procedures and still suffer.

For whom the shades on life are drawn, and you cannot see the light of day.

Table of Contents

Acknowledgements

I am not the genius, just a messenger. It was dumb luck to cross paths with Thomas Griner. In a world full of false prophets, he turned out to be the genuine article. Thomas, your work never ceases to amaze me. It has added great meaning to life. Thank you.

No small debt of gratitude goes to Karen Cassell. Her deft handling of my skepticism, and introduction to Thomas Griner showed me the light. Karen, you're an angel. Your hands are amazing and you have taught me much. Thank you.

Immeasurable gratitude goes to the undying love and support of my parents and family who have made this all possible. Thank you.

DISC SHMISC

3rd edition

a more accurate model of back pain

Introduction

Many of our currently accepted models of back pain are quite simply inaccurate. Although it appears a ruptured disc is pinching a nerve as it exits the spine on MRI, it is not. It is an innocent bystander that looks guilty, and been taking the blame for a crime it did not commit.

Did you know there is no correlation between discs and back pain? I'm not making that up, that is a conclusion in medical literature. Doctors all know this, but it's what we were raised on, and with nothing better to replace it with, it remains the diagnosis of the day, handed out as fact, but it is not a fact.

We have been stuck on disc theory for three reasons:

1. The symptoms feel nothing like a muscle.

We all know what sore muscles feel like, and this doesn't feel anything like that, this feels deadly serious. The pain feels deep in the joint, or indeed, as though a disc is pinching a nerve. The numbness and tingling down your leg feel nothing like a muscle. Right now, how you describe your symptoms has everything to do with how it will be diagnosed.

2. There is no apparent spasm

"In the thousands of patients I have examined through the years I have rarely found the involved muscles to be in spasm." Dr John Sarno, author of the book 'Healing back pain, the mind body connection.' In the vast majority of cases there is no apparent spasm.

3. What else could it be?

It is assumed muscles heal as a broken bone would. Thus, when pain becomes chronic and fails to resolve with all manner of conservative and muscle therapy - what else could it be?

The basis of back pain is a muscle problem. At the moment it is diagnosed as a herniated disc, sciatica, arthritis, stenosis, spondylolisthesis, a bone spur, etc. In truth, the problem is an underlying spasm pattern that is missed or not treated correctly. And it's very understandable – there is no apparent spasm, but that's where the source of pain is hiding.

Consider your muscles a patch of grass: you can go over the grass with a steamroller. Lean on it. Ice it. Heat it. Electrocute it. Cut it. Stretch it. Fertilize it. Pet it. Talk to it. Shine a white light on it. Can we all agree they all have a different effect on the grass than if we simply took a leaf rake to it?

Thus many treatments claim to treat your muscles, but they do not have the same effect. They may have the same intention, but they do not have the same effect, and this is why they don't work on tough cases. There's a better way to treat muscles and it solves the mystery of back pain. I call it Advanced Muscle Reconditioning, or AMR. AMR establishes historic principles and guidelines that redefine muscle therapy, and reveal the true source of pain and dysfunction.

Right now, the world of spine medicine is very confusing, overflowing with experts, gurus and opinions. Why? Because everything works some times. For 80% of the population suffering back pain, it doesn't matter who they see, or what type of treatment they get - it all works. Thus, everyone's a genius, everyone has a fan club, and I'm not here to debate anyone's experience. But for 20% pain becomes chronic, and it's half of those, 10% that are on a slippery slope heading toward surgery, because nothing is working and life is miserable. These 10% are the entire basis of my thesis. The tough cases: when cortisone, chiropractic, physical therapy, acupuncture, stretching, core strengthening and various forms of deep muscle therapy have all come up short.

In the process of fixing tough cases, variously diagnosed as a disc, arthritis, stenosis, spondylolisthesis, a bone spur, etc., we get the holy grail, the entire purpose of orthopedic-neurological examination, which is to recreate the familiar pain the patient has been suffering. To hear the patient say, *That's it. That's my problem.* You might not get that on the first visit, but definitely during the process, its what I'm looking for as I treat. My friends, *that's it,* is what doctors look for in examination – yet do not find. When we go to school, we learn early on that most of the time you can go through the entire exam and not get that. Current day diagnoses are merely an attempt to account for symptoms. This is a watershed moment in spine medicine, and I invite my colleagues in the field of spine medicine to peer review my work.

Like the game of golf, AMR is elegant in its simplicity, despite the difficulty to do it well, and so tapped in that civilians with no prior experience will be amazed at the results they can achieve.

When it comes to back pain, we'll look back on this period as the dark ages. What were we thinking? And, what took so long to figure this out? Hindsight is always 20/20.

Disc Shmisc

People often come to me convinced a disc is pinching a nerve, their doctor showed it to them right there on MRI, and what can I possibly do about that? It's simple, the disc is irrelevant. It only appears the disc is pinching a nerve. You haven't heard the whole story.

Disc history

Discs are the pads between adjacent vertebrae of the spine. Like a jelly doughnut, the center of the disc is filled with a jelly like substance. This jelly center is surrounded by fibrous tissue like the rings of a tree trunk. When a tear develops through the rings from the center to the outside, it creates a path, allowing the jelly to ooze out like so much toothpaste at the end of the tube.

DISC SHMISC

Years ago, all we had were x-rays. X-rays can only look at bone, you cannot see the disc itself. But because the space between bones, where the disc would be, looked degenerated or narrowed, we would surmise that the disc was bad, and this was the cause of your symptoms.

With the advent of magnetic resonance imaging, MRI, we could actually see the disc itself, and aha! A herniated disc! As we always suspected. And it looks for all the world as though it is pinching the nerve as it exits the spine - finally, the smoking gun. But, with more research, more and more conflicting evidence kept coming forward.

- MRI's were taken of people who never in their lives had an incidence of back pain, and guess what they found? Herniated discs.

- The disc can herniate to the left, looks like it's pinching the nerve that travels down the left leg – but the pain goes down the right leg.

- Herniated discs routinely shrink or disappear on subsequent MRI, all on their own – yet symptoms remain.

Disc Shmisc

- Half the population over age forty, has a herniated disc, or other defect deemed significant on x-ray or MRI – yet they are not in pain.

- In fact, it's not a question anymore, rather a conclusion: there is no correlation between discs and back pain.

"There was not a clear relationship between the MRI appearance of the lumbar spine and LBP. (low back pain) Thirty-two percent of asymptomatic subjects had 'abnormal' lumbar spines and 47% of all the subjects who had experienced LBP had 'normal' lumbar spines." Eur Spine J. 1997;6(2):106-14.

"However, significant proportions of asymptomatic subjects have disc herniation and neural compromise. Whilst neural compromise may be the best radiological feature distinguishing patients who may benefit from intervention, it cannot predict quality of life deficits in the diffuse group of patients with LBP." Eur Spine J. 1998;7(5):369-75

"There was no relationship between herniation type, size, and behavior over time with outcome. CONCLUSION: In typical patients with LBP or radiculopathy, MR imaging does not appear to have measurable value in terms of planning conservative care." Radiology. 2005 Nov;237(2):597-604.

With nothing better to replace it with, doctors are merely handing out a theory that has been handed down to them for generations. You go to a doctor for answers, not to hear, "I don't know," or "We're not sure." They know the hard evidence makes no sense, but they have nothing better to replace it with, so they continue to hand out this flawed theory as though it were fact. Before I knew better, I did the same.

* * *

Most doctors would never admit this to you, but you can go through the entire orthopedic-neurological examination: x-ray, MRI, range of motion, reflexes, sensation testing, orthopedic tests, palpation etc., and still not be able to put a finger on where the pain is coming from.

In an expose' on back surgery, *A knife in the back*, *The New Yorker*, April '02, the author gets orthopedic surgeons, sometimes speaking on the condition of anonymity, to admit it:

Disc Shmisc

"When I began in spine there were a handful of fellowships in the country. There are now over eighty fellowship programs in spine surgery. That means each year more and more specialists are being trained . . . We have new toys to play with – all sorts of screws, rods, and cages. And at the same time, we still don't have a clue where the pain is coming from in the vast majority of chronic sufferers."

"If you have a screwdriver, everything looks like a screw . . . There will be a lot of people doing the wrong thing for back pain for a long time, until we finally figure it out. I just hope that we don't hurt too many people in the process."

"In medicine, if you are able to stick a needle into a person, you are reimbursed at a much better rate by the insurance company. So there is a tremendous drive to perform invasive procedures. At the hospital where I was a fellow training in 1993, discograms were rarely done . . . over the last few years they have come into vogue. Surgeons and others order them routinely.

Discography (discograms)

Often there is more than one herniated disc, and whether it's profit, or they really don't know which one they want to operate on, a procedure called discography is performed.

DISC SHMISC

A needle is pressed through the muscles into the edge of each disc with increasing amounts of pressure, in an effort to reproduce the familiar pain the patient has been suffering.

Like the herniated disc, it is sold as cut and dried science, yet research findings on discography are also conflicting. There are people in pain, who have no pain on the procedure. There are people that have no pain, but do have pain on the procedure. So what does it mean? Not much, except as noted above, there is a tremendous drive to perform invasive procedures.

* * *

This conflicting evidence regarding back pain has caused many doctors to conclude it's all in your head. Dr John Sarno, a famous medical doctor on the east coast, proposes this theory in his book, *Healing Back Pain, the mind-body connection."*

In his book he shares his frustration treating large volumes of patients with neck, shoulder, back and buttock pain – *one could never predict the outcome.* And the troubling realization that the examination findings often did not correlate with the pattern of pain, ie., a disc that's herniated to the left, but the pain traveled down the right leg.

Disc Shmisc

Dr Sarno then concludes that since the hard evidence of back pain makes no sense, pain must therefore be all in your head, the result of repressed emotions, and anger. His cure? Knowledge. That the pain is all in your head.

Here's a partial list of his daily reminders:

"The pain is due to TMS, not to a structural abnormality."

"I will shift my attention from the pain to emotional issues."

"I will not be concerned or intimidated by the pain."

"TMS is a harmless condition caused by repressed emotions."

"The principle emotion is my repressed anger."

"I must think psychological at all times, not physical."

He also writes: *"In the tradition of scientific medicine I invite my colleagues to verify or correct my work."* And here's the missing link:

"In the thousands of patients I have examined through the years I have rarely found the involved muscles to be in spasm."

That is it! What we've all been missing. The underlying spasm pattern. It's quite understandable, nothing sticks out. There is no apparent spasm, but that's where the source of your pain is hiding.

Typical forms of deep muscle therapy work at times but are unable to fix tough cases. They are gross, over pressing and lack the refinement necessary to unravel advanced spasm patterns.

* * *

It is assumed muscles heal much as a broken bone would. When pain becomes chronic, there's no apparent spasm, and it fails to resolve with all manner of muscle therapy, we're left scratching our heads — must be a disc. We know the hard evidence makes no sense, but what else could it be? Thus, at this moment disc theory remains a snap judgement:

If you have a herniated disc and have no pain, it is said to be asymptomatic, or not causing symptoms. But, if you are in pain and a herniated disc is seen, you can be sure it will be blamed on the disc.

I submit to you, the disc is irrelevant. It's not whether the disc is symptomatic or not, it's whether your muscles are symptomatic or not.

8

Disc Shmisc

I understand, when your back goes out, it does not feel like just a muscle. Me telling you it's a muscle goes against your intuition. Yet, science teaches us that many things go against our intuition:

- At one point in history it seemed quite obvious the earth was flat. We now have every confidence it is round.

- It was once thought only logical to assume the sun revolved around the earth. We now know the earth spins and revolves around the sun.

We take these truths for granted, but these were revolutionary concepts for their time. At this moment, this is a revolutionary concept.

And here's the clincher: Remember the point of discography? To reproduce the familiar pain the patient has been suffering? That is the entire purpose of orthopedic-neurological examination, and that is exactly what we do every time we fix a "disc" case. Every time I fix a disc case, it doesn't matter the size or the location, without fail, at some point in the process, the patient will exclaim, *That's it! That's my problem,* and it's nowhere near a disc, it's in the muscles!

DISC SHMISC
A Landmark Case

I can hear you now, *Are you saying a disc never pinches a nerve? Would you not agree it's possible, a large herniated disc could pinch a nerve?* I would have said yes, until Danny came through my door.

Danny was a 30 year-old actor when he first hurt his low back doing a fight scene in a commercial. Entangled in wrestling maneuvers, his low back went out. The nurse on the set assured him he'd be ok, and that he need not go to the hospital. He couldn't walk for a week, and like an old man for a couple more. Being a tough guy, he never sought treatment, took ibuprofen here and there, and over the course of several months the pain subsided.

Several months later he was snow skiing. It was the end of the day, his legs were a little tired, but you know, one more run. He went over a jump when his back went out again, only this time he also felt radiating pain down the leg, numbness and tingling into the testicles, and pain on urination. This, of course, will send a guy to the doctor.

Knowing his sexual history, he knew it couldn't be an STD, nonetheless, he thought it best to see a doctor and rule out venereal disease. When the doctor learned he had recently hurt his back he said, "Oh, I know what this is, I think it's a disc".

He recommended he see a physical therapist first, before getting an MRI. He said no surgeon would operate with an MRI older than four months. "So try the physical therapy first, if that doesn't work, you can get the MRI, and go straight to surgery."

He went to physical therapy but things kept getting worse. "I'd be in the office, and my mind would tell me I'm getting treatment, so this must be good. And some of the stretches and things would seem to alleviate some of the tightness. But I would go home, or go to work, and I would feel increasingly sore, and even more tight. My flexibility seemed to be diminished, the more I went to physical therapy."

One day, "They decided to do a stretch on me, to help alleviate the pressure on the disc, as they say, right after they had done ultrasound and ice packs. My back went out on the table, in the physical therapist's hands. It felt worse than before. I fell to the floor, couldn't stand, I'm in the middle of this office, and after about 20 minutes of lying on the floor, I got up and waddled to my car. And I thought, this can't be good. Maybe I do need surgery. Maybe the doctor was right."

DISC SHMISC

An MRI was taken showing a herniated disc. The physician suggested he go back to physical therapy, but Danny wanted to try chiropractic.

He got a referral to a chiropractor who had a reputation for fixing stunt people. It would be up and down; moments when it felt good, moments when it felt bad, until it started going downhill. Not only did he have numbness, pain on urination, symptoms in his leg, back, and groin, but the symptoms increased, and he started having stomach problems. He was getting worried. From all that he'd read and what doctors were telling him, if he let this go on it could cause permanent nerve damage.

"One night I woke and was in so much pain. I got into all fours on the floor, and it literally felt like, I have no other way of describing this, someone was taking a knife and sticking it right up through my penis. And I thought, something is wrong here. This cannot be my back. This has to be something else. So I went back to the doctor, told him what was going on. He ran some tests, everything else is fine. 'This is 100% attributed to your disc, and you must go see a surgeon'."

Instead, he went back to the chiropractor, he tried acupuncture, and did the physical therapy exercises, but nothing seemed to be working.

Disc Shmisc

One night the pain was so severe he got up and went to a friend's house asking for help. Through their connections they got him in to see the founding director of the spine institute at Cedars-Sinai in Los Angeles. The expert's expert, and doctor to the stars.

The doctor looks at the MRI and is surprised to see a large protrusion at L5-S1 that was nearly occluding the entire spinal canal. "This is a really bad MRI. This is not good. I think you have Cauda Equina Syndrome*, or the beginnings of it."

* The spinal chord itself ends at around the level of the second lumbar vertebrae and turns into a horse tail of nerve roots, or "cauda equina," that travel the remaining distance in the spinal canal, and then exit between vertebrae at their respective levels. Thus chord compression at the L5-S1 level is called compression of the cauda equina.

Surgery was deemed imperative – that disc was pinching the lower end of his spinal chord, and the nerves leading into his testicles. Surgery was scheduled, but workers compensation insurance refused to pay for it.

He was thus sent for review to the workers comp doctor who said:

DISC SHMISC

"Danny, it's my job to defend workers comp and say you don't need this surgery, but I agree with your doctor. You have one of the worst MRI's I've ever seen. If you have 13 mm of space for the spinal chord it's considered a surgical emergency. Danny, you don't have 13 mm, you have 5 mm. You could literally sneeze and go paralyzed for life. You must have this surgery." This is the guy defending workers comp. Who would question this?

Danny had researched the medical literature and found that discs can shrink or disappear on subsequent MRI, all on their own. He had spoken with enough people that had back surgery to find it was no panacea, and to be avoided if at all possible. He knew the MRI they were going on was pretty old now and some things didn't make sense, for example, he was able to touch his toes. To satisfy his own curiosity before having major back surgery at 30 years of age, he requested another MRI. The workers comp doctor says, "You don't need another MRI." "Can't things change?" "They can but yours is a really bad situation. You have to have surgery." Danny insisted on, and got, a second MRI.

He returns to consult with the director of the spine institute on the results of the second MRI. The doctor greets him and says, "Congratulations! You must be feeling better. The disc herniation is greatly reduced*, surgery is no longer necessary."

14

Disc Shmisc

* In fact, the large protrusion at L5-S1 had disappeared, looking completely normal. Now there was a small bulge at L4-5.

Danny says, "Really? To be honest I still feel the same. You mean you don't know what's causing my symptoms?"

He says, "Well, there could be some enzymes released" . . . , but before he leaves, the doctor divulged, "Danny, what you need to know about my profession – there are absolutely no certainties."

This confirmed for Danny what his experience had been — that doctors operate from a series of educated guesses. There are very few absolutes, particularly in the area of the spine. Yet for the preservation of the industry, and to alleviate people's fear, the presentation is, we know what we're talking about. The reality is quite the opposite.

Danny then found me. I'd come to understand some time ago a typical herniated disc was nothing more than a muscle pull to a weight bearing joint. But one of this size? Even I thought surely this would pinch a nerve. And numbness into the testicles? That was a new one.

DISC SHMISC

We're all the same and we're all different, each person, you figure them out. Fixing tough cases is not magic, it's technique and hard work. We discovered a spasm pattern into the groin and as I worked it he exclaimed, "That's it, that's what's causing the tingling into my testicles." At some point we broke through the pattern in his low back and he said, "That's it, that's the original injury to my low back." With this work we put you in touch with exactly what the problem is, and it's nowhere near a disc.

"The minute he laid his hands on me I knew that I had found the solution. I knew because I had experienced and tried enough things to know when something was different. And how I felt when I got off the table that first time, I had not felt that with anything else. By the end of the 8th session I was functioning as if I had not even had to go through a back disorder. I was able to walk, the pain in my leg was gone, the pain in my groin was gone, and what I realized was that, there was an answer."

If ever there was a disc that should be pinching a nerve, this was it - and it wasn't. It would appear that nerves are more like our own electrical chords, you can step on them, yet it still doesn't crimp the current going to the lamp.

Again, it's only too understandable why we have been stuck on disc theory: the symptoms feel nothing like a muscle, there's no apparent spasm, and what can you say when pain becomes chronic and fails to resolve with all manner of muscle therapy?

That's why doctors, to this day, are stuck gazing at joints and discs on x-ray and MRI as though muscles don't exist.

at this moment, what you don't know can hurt you

"Conclusions. Previous back surgery is associated with significantly worse general health status than those without surgery." SPINE Volume 29, Number 17, pp 1931-37

"Conclusion. This pilot study showed no difference between surgical or medical management for recovery or improvement in patients with discogenic paresis." SPINE Volume 27, Number 13, pp 1426-32. (discogenic paresis is muscular weakness, or partial paralysis currently thought to be the result of nerve damage from a disc)

"Low back pain persisting or appearing after a technically successful lumbar fusion challenges clinicians." Eur Spine J. 2005 Sep;14(7):654-8. Epub 2005 Mar 11.

"Conclusions. In the majority of our patients, standard decompression and fusion procedures were not 'successful.' . . . Loss of neurological function (strength, sensation, bowel and bladder control) was reported by patients more often than improvements." Neurosurgery Volume 28, No. 5 pp 685-89. Failed back surgery syndrome: 5 year follow-up in 102 patients undergoing repeated operations.

"Despite the continuous development of surgical techniques and implants, a substantial number of patients still undergo surgery for chronic low back pain without any benefit, or even become worse." Eur Spine J. 2003 Feb;12(1):22-33. Epub 2002 Oct 23.

"Since that time spinal surgery has witnessed an industrial explosion, resulting in a multibillion dollar industry. . . . consider the 'fusion cage explosion.' In the year after the 1996 approval of the BK and Ray cages, sales in excess of $100 million were realized. Four years later the efficacy of these stand alone devices is very questionable." SPINE Volume 26, Number 18, pp 1947-49 Presidential Address: Surgeons, Societies and companies: ethics and legalities.

"The surgeons themselves are guilty of being insufficiently critical of products and techniques they are developing. . . . More people are interested in getting on the gravy train than on stopping the gravy train." Dr Richard Deyo, Professor Oregon Health and Science University.

Disc Shmisc

" . . . financial conflict often skews the results of clinical and basic research toward favoring the drug or device in question." SPINE Volume 27, Number 1, pp 6-10.

Conflict of interest is a huge problem in the industry. According to Dr Robert Steinbrook, in an article in the New England Journal of Medicine, it is very likely your doctor has a tie to a company that makes a drug or device. And while doctors easily move on to the next drug or device, suffering patients are often left in their wake.

A 45 year old woman was sold on the need for an artificial disc to relieve her low back pain. "He said my back would be better than ever." She thought to herself, "Wow, disc replacement is the best thing since sliced bread." After surgery, she was in debilitating pain, able to walk only with the assistance of a walker. She had a second operation in an attempt to correct the first one. "I couldn't take enough drugs for the pain. . . . Having that surgery was the worst decision of my life."

Later, she was "livid" when she found out her surgeon had financial ties to the company making the artificial disc.

Failed Back Surgery Syndrome

It's called "failed back surgery syndrome," or FBSS, when surgery fails to relieve pain or makes you worse. The July '04 issue of *The Back Letter*, contains the following indictment: "The world of spinal medicine, unfortunately, is producing patients with failed back surgery syndrome at an alarming rate." Volume 12, No. 7 pp 79

All this begs the question: why does surgery ever work at all? Perhaps by cutting through the muscles and putting some slack in the system.

Example: *Male, 50's, he's had 4 disc surgeries. After the fourth one he says he's had sciatica every day since. He didn't come to me for this however, he came in for treatment of numbness and tingling in his hands as he worked doing carpentry. After a number of sessions working his arms, hands and neck he tells me that since I started working on him his sciatica has completely disappeared. And I've not touched him below the level of his shoulder blade!*

That's not my normal approach to sciatica. What to make of it? I call it putting slack in the system. Our muscles are all connected, just as one freeway leads to another. By putting slack anywhere in the system, it can help the system as a whole.

Disc Shmisc

It has also been shown that surgery is most successful on the young, whose muscles are at their most resilient, and able to compensate.

* * *

A good theory is able to account for all, or most of the relevant facts, and is not contradicted by any of them. It is obvious, disc theory no longer meets this criteria. The disc is not the problem. The posse is off track.

Surgeons, through no fault of their own, are operating, literally, on a flawed premise.

The latest in technologies, such as artificial discs, are doomed to failure, and early returns are already in. Surgeon Andre van Ooij of the Netherlands, who has observed a significant number of post artificial disc implants in Europe said in a letter to the Editor of the North American Spine Society publication, SpineLine: "These patients represent the most disabled group of patients that I have personally seen in 24 years of spine practice."

* * *

DISC SHMISC

Disc theory was the consensus of scholarly thought well before the advent of MRI. Most every textbook on anatomy will take time to illustrate how a disc can pinch a nerve. The concept has been seared upon our consciousness for generations. With the emergence of MRI, doctors know the hard evidence makes no sense, yet with nothing better to replace it with, it remains the diagnosis of the day. It is time to put disc theory out to pasture with other outdated theories.

Arthritis

When you look at an x-ray without a patient history to go with it, you cannot tell whether or where a person is in pain. There are exceptions, but in general this is true. This is why a patient history, describing the location of pain, accompanies every x-ray to be read by the radiologist.

You could look at the most perfectly normal healthy spine on x-ray, and that person could be in acute pain. Conversely, you could see the most severely degenerated joint on x-ray, but there is no complaint of pain there whatsoever.

If you see an arthritic joint and there is no complaint of pain, it is said to be asymptomatic, or not causing symptoms. But, if you are in pain and they see an arthritic joint, you can be sure it will be blamed on arthritis.

I submit to you, the arthritis is irrelevant. It's not whether the arthritic joint is symptomatic or not, it's whether your muscles are symptomatic or not.

Severe Arthritis / Scoliosis

Early in my career, I had a 68 year old woman, who had the most degenerated, scoliotic spine I've ever seen. Ideally your spine, when viewed from in front or behind, is nice and straight like this letter "I." Her spine was literally shaped like this "S." When I saw it on x-ray I was shocked. My gut reaction was, she should get her affairs in order. I didn't know how she could be alive and walking around with such a thing. It was so severely degenerated, you couldn't see any way possible for a nerve to exit the spine. She had numbness and tingling into her right hand, and was on medication for chronic low back pain.

I would have sent her away thinking surely there was nothing we could do for her, but was working for another chiropractor at the time who said to have a little faith and give it a go. She was a very sweet and loyal patient, and guess what? It helped. Although we could never get the tingling out of her thumb, and she still required medication for chronic low back pain, she felt some degree of relief and kept returning for treatment.

With a spine like that, what do you expect? We worked regularly for two years, I threw many techniques at her until treatments just weren't doing anything and I said, "You know, I just don't think there is anything more we can do for you." Some time later, after crossing paths with Thomas Griner, I called her back and said I was very impressed with this man's work, and thought it might offer some benefit. We did weekly hour sessions over the course of a year, only this time we were able to get all of the numbness and tingling out of her right hand – including the thumb. It gave her such relief she stopped taking medications for chronic low back pain. I couldn't believe it. You can bet her spine was still completely degenerated and scoliotic, yet her pain and tingling went away

What else can you conclude except arthritis pain is actually the result of an underlying spasm pattern crimping the joint? When treated correctly, and you release the vice-like grip of spasm, the joint can breath again, and pain is eliminated from even the most severely degenerated joints. You can get away with what I consider over pressing forms of massage when muscles are young and resilient, but they don't work on tough cases, and older crusty muscles.

DISC SHMISC
Bone on Bone Arthritis

A man in his 80's told me this story: His right hip had been bothering him for several years, until it got so bad he went to the doctor. He said "Interestingly enough, on x-ray, the other hip was more arthritic." Yet, it was his less arthritic hip that was bothering him. He received a shot of cortisone and it was miraculous. He said he stumbled into the doctor's office, and walked out.

A year later he felt something tweak in the same right hip. He didn't think much of it at the moment, but after waking from a nap there was a sharp jabbing nerve pain piercing the right hip and groin. This time however, cortisone did not do the trick, and surgery was recommended for, "bone on bone" arthritis.

Remember, a year ago, x-rays showed his other hip to be more arthritic. I told him if he gave me a chance I'd prove to him he didn't need a hip replacement.

After two hour-and-a-half sessions we hadn't made a dent. He felt bruised and beaten up from me working on him, and no better. After the third session however, we started making progress, and

Arthritis

after ten sessions he came in one day and said there was no reason for him to be there, his hip felt fine.

I'm at a social event and a man in his 60's relates this story. He loves to play golf, and walks the course with no problem. One day he is on a ladder cleaning out the eaves on his house, when reaching, he feels something tweak in his hip. The hip freezes up on him, and the doctor says he needs a hip replacement for "bone on bone arthritis." You don't go from walking 18 holes one day to needing a hip replacement the next. He was scheduled for surgery and didn't want to hear an opposing opinion. Showing someone an arthritic joint on x-ray is an easy sell, and appears a logical conclusion, but it is far from the whole story. In replacing the hip joint they slice through every muscle attaching to it, and this may be the reason it sometimes relieves pain.

Two things you need to know about back pain.

1. What's the number one axiom of back pain?

It's self-limiting.

Back pain, by definition, is what we call self-limiting. Meaning if you do nothing, it will normally go away on its own in a reasonable amount of time.

When young, we expect pain to go away with a little rest. When pain doesn't go away, we seek help. When pain is disrupting every aspect of life for six months to a year, and fails to resolve with all manner of therapy, most people are at the end of their rope, and susceptible to the surgeon's advice. Yet the principle remains: if you did nothing long enough, and quit aggravating it, it would eventually die down to a dull roar, it will just take much longer than most people can handle. And when it does, you may not be the person you used to be.

Two things you need to know about back pain

Example 1. *Jim, 60's, hurt his low back in 2000. While changing a tire he felt something tweak, resulting in acute low back pain radiating into the legs.*

An MRI showed a sequestered disc at L2-3. A sequestered disc is one where the jelly has squirted out and separated from the parent material. (think of the toothpaste on your brush, separate from the tube)

Jim is a little unique in that he sought the advice of some twenty doctors, including ten orthopedic surgeons, and five neurosurgeons. Ninety percent of them recommended surgery. They were sure that sequestered disc was pressing on a nerve causing his pain. Only two, one being Dr Robert Bray, a neurosurgeon at Cedars-Sinai in Los Angeles, recommended against surgery. He said that with time, the body might break down and dissolve that sequestered disc.

Ten months later, sure enough, a new MRI revealed the sequestered disc had, indeed, disappeared. Yet he still had lingering symptoms. At that point Dr Bray deemed his spine unstable and recommended surgery to fuse the spine. Of course, Jim again sought the advice of many, who said his spine didn't look that bad and recommended against fusion, a woefully unsuccessful form of surgery. He never did have surgery, and felt protective of his spine for a long time so as not to aggravate. Indeed, in time, the pain died down, so long as he doesn't try to do too much, like play tennis. He can't be as physically active as he'd like, but he can go about his daily activities without difficulty

Example 2. Even chronic recurrent pain is self-limiting

Pat was in his thirties when he first hurt his low back, wrenching as a diesel mechanic. While stiff and sore, he could still walk and was back to work in a week. A week or so later he was trying to change a tire when it went out a second time, only this time it was much worse. "It felt as if you ripped a piece of paper in two all the way to the middle of my back. I was hunched over for 6 weeks until I could stand up straight." Muscle relaxers were no help. Twelve weeks of physical therapy didn't do much good. Doctors told him it was torn muscles and a bulging disc.

Surgery was recommended but Pat would not agree to it. When the doctor finally realized he would not be swayed, he told him that in time he might gradually heal up to 80% of what he used to be.

He never could resume work, and workers compensation considered him disabled. It was very unstable for years. "I could bend over to pick up a wash cloth and it would go out. The wind could blow the wrong way and it would go out. At the chiropractor's office, it would go out on the way out the door."

Two things you need to know about back pain

He couldn't work for four years, and then was able to do light work that didn't require bending or heavy lifting.

"It took me a long time to come back, I still ain't all the way back. It has a compressed feeling. If I pick something up that's too heavy it could still go out on me. If I went out and over exerted myself it could go out and lay me up for a week or two. Twenty years, a little at a time, it's gotten better, and I've gotten wiser and learned my limits. I quit over exerting it. Maybe I would have come back quicker if I took it easy all the time, but I had two boys growing up."

He had one episode that is worth mentioning as it would have sent many straight to surgery: "A couple years ago I had a pain through the cheek of my [butt], clear down through the knee to the toe. Just woke up with it one day. It ached all the way to my little toe. First time I ever had that. My back has hurt into the hips but never through the leg. My knee ached. I wasn't right for at least six months. Adjustments didn't help. My back didn't hurt, it was just below the belt, from my cheek down the leg. Then one day I was unloading a boat and felt it snap, and it felt better. Instant relief. I felt sore for a few days, but it had realigned itself. I was taking Alieve every 3-4 hours."

"It hasn't gone out much the last couple years. Up until then probably 3-4 times a year depending on how much screwing around I did. I've gotten wiser and stopped trying to do things that would make it go out."

"I'm glad I never had surgery. Everyone I know whose had surgery is worse off than I am. I have a buddy of mine who fell on the ice. He went right to a specialist, now he's on his third disc surgery."

2. Everything works sometimes.

For 80% of the population suffering back pain, it doesn't matter who they see, or what type of treatment they get, it all works. That's why there are ten thousand gurus out there right now claiming to have the answer to back pain. Everyone and their cousin has their guru that fixed them. I'm not here to dispute anyone's experience.

But for 20%, pain becomes chronic, and it's half of those, 10%, that are on a slippery slope heading toward surgery because nothing is working and life is miserable. Everything I'm telling you comes from the 10%, when surgery was thought to be the only remaining option.

Two things you need to know about back pain

Here's a classic example: *A man, 50's, tells me his low back first went out on him 15 years ago. Chiropractic and physical therapy had fixed him up fine. Fifteen years later his back goes out again. Only this time a year of physical therapy and chiropractic wasn't getting the job done. He estimated 35 bad weeks to 15 good ones in the year prior. Life was miserable and he was unable to play golf.*

Some regular hour-long sessions with me, and he is pain free, playing golf, and holding stable. Haven't seen him in years.

A more accurate model of back pain

This is your spine. (picture a spine upright, nice and straight)

This is your spine without muscles. (picture bones lying in a heap on the floor)

Bones give us shape so we're not blobs oozing about, but bones do not move anywhere on their own. Bones are held up and in suspension by muscles. You move because muscles move you.

Ideally your spine looks like this:

- nice and straight when viewed from behind, or in front.

A more accurate model of back pain

- from the side, a curve in the low back and neck, and a hump in the middle.

This is a nice ideal, but rarely does anyone have such a spine. Most all of us are crooked and always have been. Our muscles pick up this crooked, imperfect thing, and run with it as though we are superman or wonderwoman for many years. When you're in pain, it's not because you're spine is crooked, it always has been. It's because the muscles that support your crooked spine had a breakdown.

How strong are muscles?

Many people carry around congenital deformities for decades and have no clue they exist. I had a woman with a congenital deformity where only one half of the lowest vertebrae in her spine had formed. Yet she was a dancer and in her 40's when her low back went out for the first time.

When you're in pain, it's not because of a congenital deformity, it's because the muscles supporting your congenital deformity had a breakdown.

There is a condition called spondylolisthesis, I'll call it spondylo for short, where there is a fracture allowing the front part of the vertebrae, or body, to separate and slip forward to varying degrees from the back part, or articular portion of the vertebrae. It looks completely dislocated and horrifying on x-ray. Yet people play football, and are active with these things for years and have no awareness of their existence.

I have a friend in his 50's who has one. He's had episodes of pain with long periods of stability, yet whenever his back goes out it's blamed on the spondylo. But if the spondylo has been there all along, why isn't he in pain all along? Because the muscles that pick up the spondylo and run with it are holding stable. When you're in pain, it's not because of a spondylo, it's because the muscles supporting the spondylo had a breakdown.

Anatomy of a muscle

Each individual muscle fiber contains numerous contractile elements, and is wrapped in a fibrous, saran-wrap-like connective tissue. Groups of fibers are wrapped into bundles. Bundles are wrapped together to make a muscle belly. This connective tissue saran wrap, from the fiber, to the bundle, to the belly, is contiguous with the tendon which attaches to bone, or to another tendon. Muscles are saran wrapped individually and in groups for support, and to help direct their action. Groups of muscles are wrapped together making us a whole. Giving us the shape and form of our bodies, and a container for its contents. This saran wrap also connects skin to muscle. As you can see, this connective tissue saran wrap is very integrated. Once you put the sauce on the spaghetti, how do you separate?* The only distinction I'll make is the wrapping between muscles as it helps explain some things, but more on that later. (*sauce = saran wrap, or fascia. spaghetti = muscles)

36

A more accurate model of back pain

Muscles start out in life a plump juicy hot dog and slowly age into crispy bacon.

Think of your muscles as so much spaghetti. You know if you put too much spaghetti in a pot of boiling water how some of it clumps together? This is what happens to muscles, and in truth, I am just a glorified de-clumper. Muscles form underlying spasm, or clumped pasta, and we are not aware of it. It is numbed out of our awareness, a natural part of the aging process.

You can buy a new car, drive it 100,000 miles and never have a break down, but it still has 100,000 miles on it.

Same with our bodies: we may remain active and stable for years, improve strength and flexibility, and all the while clumped pasta exists and continues to form, a natural part of the aging process.

Some people may be fortunate, their muscles, like an old tire bald of tread but still rolling, may age gracefully, having never suffered a blow out.

Thus, as research shows, there are many who have never suffered back pain, yet have herniated discs on MRI. The disc is irrelevant, they never suffered back pain because their muscles aged gracefully, having never suffered a breakdown.

There are ten thousand shades of grey between hot dog and bacon, and we may be pain free and holding stable at any one of them. Each of us is a geological dig of everything that has ever happened to us.

When you see degenerated joints and discs on x-ray and MRI, think of the degenerated muscles you cannot see.

It is the slightest injury to muscle fibers, or the aggravation of underlying spasm patterns, that is the basis of back pain.

Reactive spasm / over-contraction

Muscles, even at rest, have some degree of contraction in them, this is called muscle tone, and muscle tone is considered normal. While much of muscular contraction is under our voluntary control by the brain, muscle tone is controlled by a circuit local to the spinal chord.

A more accurate model of back pain

(Guyton's physiology, 7th edition: "It is believed that skeletal muscle tone results entirely from nerve impulses coming from the spinal chord.")

When muscle fibers are injured, muscles around the injury go into a reactive contraction that is energized by reverberations in this circuit local to the spinal chord. It is beyond our ability to control. It is as if the muscles around the injury say to the brain, "Hey! We don't care if we ever work for you again, we are going to protect our own!"

It is this reactive contraction that is the basis of back pain. The disc is irrelevant, an innocent bystander that looks guilty and been taking the blame for a crime it did not commit. I postulate that it is the reactive spasm crimping on discs that causes the inner jelly to squirt out. As we so often observe, ruptured discs shrink or disappear on subsequent MRI, the body breaks down and absorbs the disc material, yet symptoms remain.

I know, when your back goes out it does not feel like a muscle pull. When you pull a surface muscle we can identify it as muscular. When you pull a muscle in direct support of a weight bearing joint, it's more like an earthquake. Those deep electric jolts of nerve pain feel deadly serious, and nothing as simple as a muscle pull, but that's what it is – reactive spasm gripping the joint.

DISC SHMISC
Sciatica is another obsolete diagnosis

Radiating pain and tingling is a result of the spasm pattern itself, or the nerve is pinched as it travels through the reactive spasm of muscle - it is not pinched by a disc as it exits the spine.

It is cliché to call any radiating pain in the low back sciatica. It's how we're taught, I used to do it myself. Any radiating pain, numbness or tingling into the glute or down the leg is automatically given the catchall diagnosis - sciatica. Yet, when I roll a portion of the iliotibial band and the patient says, "That's it," it's nowhere near the sciatic nerve. The pain is radiating along a spasm pattern.

Radiating pain or tingling into the calf and foot is simply underlying spasm there, it is not sciatica. Our feet and calves take a beating, and the pain is simply aggravated underlying spasm. It feels like a nerve, but it's caused by a muscle.

Onset

There are two classic modes to the onset of pain. Sometimes the tweak is so minor, you don't notice anything. What you notice is increasing stiffness that sets in over time, until the grip of contraction has you locked up in pain.

Other times you go straight to the ground with a sharp jabbing nerve pain that one woman compared to childbirth. If it's never

A more accurate model of back pain

happened to you before, it can be most frightening. You can't imagine ever being able to walk normally again. Life stops in its tracks. The pain is an energy sink, draining your body of its mojo. You will consistently find these people irritable, with a shorter fuse than normal.

If you do nothing, given enough time the reverberating circuit energizing the reactive spasm dies down, and the grip fades away.

Yet muscles do not completely heal from injury. Some fibers remain hypertonic, or too tight even at rest. The nerves that would inform the brain of pain and spasm numb out. There is residual hypertonicity, or underlying spasm, and you are not aware of it.

There forms a combination of hypertonic muscle (muscle contracting more than normal, even at rest), and an actual clumping of the connective tissue saran wrap — clumped pasta.

* * *

Thus, your muscles form clumped pasta as a natural result of the aging process, and more significantly, as the lingering effect of injury.

DISC SHMISC

When young, we're used to pain going away with a little rest. Your muscles make a little bacon and you're right as rain. Young muscles are fleshy, resilient, and able to compensate. Every treatment works. However, not every treatment reconditions your muscles, many treatments just help numb pain and spasm out of your awareness, which is what your body would do on its own.

When I roll your muscles, and you say, "Wow, what's that? I didn't know that was there," that is underlying spasm that has been numbed out of your awareness.

In so many cases, as I scout other areas of the body I find very advanced spasm patterns — had they told me they were in pain there, I would have believed them. Yet, they never complained of pain there, their bacon was holding stable.

I can put you in touch with spasm all over your body, that you had no idea existed, and may cause you no pain. I can't tell which ones are symptomatic, I simply ask where it hurts. It's like an itch, and only you know where it wants to be scratched.

It is the reactive spasm from injury that is not reconditioned properly and leads to chronic pain, and a feeling something isn't right. Patients can often relate their pain to an old injury, and not

A more accurate model of back pain

being the same since, or getting progressively worse. They haven't had their muscles treated right.

* * *

When you're young and you tweak a muscle, there is a hard knot of reactive spasm that sticks out like a sore thumb, and it's obvious - that's a muscle spasm. With age, and in so many chronic cases, nothing sticks out, there is no apparent spasm. Like the folds of an accordion, muscle fibers pleat together as though they were never there, but that's where the source of your pain is hiding.

Because there is no apparent spasm, because the pain feels like a nerve, or deep in the joint, and because historically muscle therapy fails to resolve chronic cases, doctors to this day diagnose strictly by what they see on x-ray and MRI. Even though they know there is no correlation between the hard evidence and back pain. It's simply a matter of, if you're in pain, this must be what's causing it.

When an acute episode of pain subsides, maybe you go back to aging gracefully. For many, stretching and strengthening does wonders. Maybe you instinctively limit your activities so as not to aggravate. You're no spring chicken anymore, what do you expect? These clumped underlying patterns do not have the physical ability to perform as healthy muscle would. Maybe you feel no pain going about daily life, but these areas do not hold up to the demands of your favorite activity.

Ever notice how arthritis pain flares up from overuse? The arthritic joint is irrelevant, it's from overusing your degenerated muscles, aggravating the underlying pattern.

If your injury is serious enough, or you set off an aged underlying pattern, you could be in for a long road of trouble, as therapies that used to work so well no longer get the job done. It will take a long time for one of these patterns to numb out, and when it does, it's likely you won't be the person you used to be.

Is back pain all in your head?

Absolutely not. Your muscles pick up an imperfect spine and run with it for decades, yet whenever your body aches it must be all in your head? Give me a break.

Life is a combination plate. We have day and night, love and fear, mind and body. Not everything is in your head. If thoughts were so powerful we wouldn't age. If back pain is directly related to

A more accurate model of back pain

emotions, you tell me why teenagers aren't screaming with back pain – in unison. Back pain is not directly related to emotions. Emotions and stress can have deleterious effects on health, but as far as their direct effect on muscles, perhaps a miniscule amount of tension that by itself is not enough to cause any harm.

Yet Dr Sarno has a large following, and many will sing his praises, how can this be? I call it *ignoring*, or *being distracted*. It is an interesting phenomenon and maybe you've experienced it, you can be in pain, yet if there's a social event you must attend, you notice that while you are around people you are distracted from the pain. I believe this is why faith healers get their momentary healings.

Example. I have a patient right now who has undergone three unsuccessful surgeries for spinal stenosis and been living in chronic pain for seven years. He teaches an acting class, and according to him, as soon as he steps into class, he forgets about it completely. But as soon as class is over, there it is, bad as ever.

Remember Sarno's daily Reminders? Just keep ignoring the pain, and telling yourself the following: *"I will shift my attention from the pain to emotional issues." "I will not be concerned or intimidated by the pain." "I must think psychological at all times, not physical."*

DISC SHMISC

People suffering chronic pain that hasn't responded to "everything under the sun" are susceptible to believing anything. And who doesn't have issues? I've had patients suffering chronic pain who came to believe Dr Sarno completely. Yet, when their pain didn't go away, they were then torturing themselves with guilt at their inability to get rid of it. I applaud Dr Sarno for confronting the disagreement in hard evidence, and could not be more supportive in his efforts to help people release their pent up emotions and anger. Finding some inner peace is about the most important thing you can do in life. When you recondition muscles properly, you can resume that search without pain.

Example. I had a young lady, 20's, who provided some form of psychic healing. After giving a session one evening she noticed shoulder pain that continued to get worse and worse, until it was so painful it required a sling. She thought she'd picked up some "bad vibe," and was now working through emotional issues. Yet, if you dig into a patient's history, you will likely find a better explanation. In this case she had been partying. The lingering effect of many recreational drugs leaves your muscles tense, and dried out, but you have no clue – it's numbed out of your awareness. If I've been working on someone regularly and have a baseline reading on their muscles, I can tell when they've been partying. They have no awareness however, until I put them in touch with it. Right before the session, she remembered twirling her arms in big circles to loosen up. In doing so she did one of those minor tweaks where you don't notice anything at the moment. After the session, she noticed pain that became progressively worse over the course of several days. When it required a sling, she made an appointment Although her pain was acute, one half-hour session was all it took to fix, and she's been fine ever since.

If you squeezed her muscles as you would a piece of fruit, there was no apparent spasm, the underlying pattern can be so easily missed. I just have them point to where it hurts. In working the associated pattern I can sometimes tell which fibers have been irritated, but the patient always knows better than I do.

Why do muscles tweak?

We say that muscles are very unpredictable. They are living flesh, a part of the system as a whole, and influenced by a wide variety of factors. Have you been overdoing it, under-doing it, sitting for long periods. Are you tired, stressed, dehydrated. Are you fighting a virus. Is your diet out of whack. Is your colon clogged. Exposure to chemicals, drugs, recreational drugs, may all leave your muscles more susceptible to tweaking.

Thus, there are moments when one more stress to the system can be the straw that broke the camel's back. It is classic that one day you do a simple movement you do every day of your life, but today

– tweak. Regardless of the series of events that led to your muscle tweaking, once it tweaks, you want to recondition the reactive spasm properly.

Nutrition and back pain

People will come in, and someone they've seen will have them on all manner of nutrients, and they'll want to know if they should they keep taking them. Here's my question: You've been taking them for months now, you tell me, what have they done for you? Usually the results are negligible at best. There is nothing wrong with nutrients, they are good for you, but when it comes to back pain they are missing the crux of the problem – getting your muscles reconditioned properly. When they feel the effectiveness of the therapy it becomes abundantly clear.

The long road to AMR

I started out a chiropractor. There is an art to adjusting and I loved it, but excuse the pun, it's not everything it's cracked up to be. In the industry we call it pop and pray. You pop their bones and pray to god it works. Occasionally it's amazing, often it helps, and often it leaves you wanting.

Thus, many of us seek answers from any of a number of sideline techniques that surround our profession: Activator, AK, SOT, DNFT, BEST, Cox. Physical therapy modalities such as ultrasound, electrical muscle stimulation, stretching, strengthening, and various forms of deep muscle therapy. Techniques that work with energy, emotions and crystals. They say there's a little truth in everything? I say that in some things there is very little. (rim shot please.)

DISC SHMISC

There is no shortage of false prophets out there claiming their technique fills in the holes of chiropractic, and cures everything that ails you, but you find that much like chiropractic, they all helped some, but there were always those tough cases you couldn't fix.

Thus, there was a time I couldn't fix tough cases and deferred to orthopedists as the experts, having the final word on back pain. At the time, more and more conflicting evidence was coming out regarding discs, yet when pain became chronic and failed to resolve with all manner of therapy, what else could it be? Perhaps surgery was necessary. Back pain was a mystery.

We chiropractors consider ourselves experts without peer at feeling, or palpating, the flesh and we too have been missing the underlying spasm pattern. Like Dr Sarno, many chiropractors have concluded that chronic pain is all in your head.

Right out of school I worked for a chiropractor that could sell ice cubes to Eskimos and sold every patient on the need for an enormous series of treatments. The invaluable part of the experience is that we were allowed to use a wide variety of techniques. So I got to observe, and experiment with a wide variety of techniques, and have formed many opinions.

The long road to AMR

I then taught at the Cleveland Chiropractic College in Los Angeles, overseeing young doctors working on their first patients in the clinic, and experimented with techniques in private practice.

It was at the end of a long road that I came across a protégé of Thomas Griner, who was espousing the greatness of his muscle therapy. By now I'd heard it too many times: how great a technique was, how it cured everything that ailed you, and I didn't want to hear it. Besides, I'd gained an appreciation for muscles and been around the block on muscle therapies - I didn't think there was anything that radically different anyone could teach me about how to treat a muscle. My first assumption? I'm sure I already do that, or something similar.

Suffice it to say, I was wrong, the minute he touched me I knew he had something, he played my muscles as a completely different instrument. Instead of mashing with constant, or slow, heavy pressure, he manipulated skin and flesh in a most refined and precise manner. It felt remarkably deep, but I could tell he was using relatively little force as he played chords I never knew existed. I was stunned, I knew it was better than anything I was doing, though I had no idea how profound it would turn out to be.

To imitate Griner's work was to start from scratch despite all previous training. There are a few principles and then you apply it to different areas of the body. You learn it in segments. You might be good in the neck but clueless in the low back. Each area has its own intricacies.

I wasn't very good at first, but in time my hands became smarter, and it started happening, I started fixing the tough cases I couldn't fix before, seeing conditions change I once did not think possible. For example:

Partial paralysis from stroke

Les McCann, a legendary jazz piano player and singer, was around 60 years of age when he suffered a stroke on stage during one of his concerts. Afterward his right hand was partially paralyzed, stuck like a fist. His thumb could move, but his fingers were stuck in a clenched fist position. When he went back to playing piano he could vamp chords with his left hand but couldn't play with the right, so he brought in a couple other instruments to take over solos.

It had been stuck like this for four years, and he'd tried every therapy under the sun, when a mutual friend referred him in to have me take a look at it. I was speechless. I told him I had never seen anything like it and had no clue what could be done. My friend had more faith in me than I did. He said, "Do me a favor and see what you can do." And this is how I know what I know –

don't think, just work. If I thought about it, I would have said there was no way.

Ten one-hour sessions on his forearm and he walked out with his hand still stuck like a fist. It was the twelfth session when it broke free and was reborn right before our eyes. Les cried, he knew he was free at last. Of course his hand was weak and would take some time to regain strength, but we've rarely worked on it since. Les claims the fingers on his right hand are 98% resolved, and he enjoys playing piano fluidly again with both hands. "In the four years of therapy and all the therapists I had met before Dr Bronk, nothing can compare to the treatments of Dr Bronk.

Here are excerpts from an interview in Cosmik Debris Magazine, September 1999 - cosmik.com.

He returned to the stage as a leader while still limited to the use of a single finger, moved by his ever present desire to communicate the love that inspires his music.

Cosmik: *And that's all complicated by carpal tunnel...*

McCann: *I don't have that no more. All cured. I will sing the praises of, and you have to write this, Dr. Brian Bronk, a young man here in Los Angeles who has a treatment that cures things like* *that. For piano players and musicians it's beyond belief. He's saved many people from carpal tunnel operations.*

Cosmik: *I'll definitely write that, because that's great news. That can be debilitating, not only for musicians, but for writers, too.*

McCann: *You're right. Artists, painter, anybody who has that repetitive motion. And he's been my lifesaver musically. I'm totally in love with music again, and anytime I play with the band, they come over and say "Wow, we heard you man!" They see the improvement. I see the results, and can deal with the work because he's doing it because he loves me, and loves the music.*

Let's be clear about one thing - that was not carpal tunnel, his hand was partially paralyzed. It seems every area of the body has its catchall diagnosis that becomes part of the vernacular. ie., sciatica.

I've been in the woodshed the last twenty-five years practicing the craft, putting in the extra time to see what was possible when I had no idea, and often questioned what I was doing. It has been surprising and proving itself to me over and over. My conclusions are not rash, rather a series of deductions having fixed one tough case after another when, quite literally, all else had failed.

I never intended to become another talking head and join the chorus of voices claiming to have the answer to back pain. But

The long road to AMR

I'm quite sure of what I'm saying and feel a duty now to pass on what I've learned. I make a bold statement, and I'm sure it will be met with the same knee-jerk skepticism I had when I met Griner - there have been so many false prophets that have come before, it's only natural. I know you will have to prove it to yourself just as I had to, and you can, if you do the work.

I call the work AMR, short for Advanced Muscle Reconditioning. AMR is entirely my take on what I gleaned form Griner, his protégé's and my own observation. Griner and I both seek to explain what we observe clinically though we use very different terms to do it. If you compare our writings, it's apples and oranges, you may not realize we're talking about the same thing. My simplified explanation, metaphor and opinion will no doubt cause him great suffering, but it is Griner's influence that set me straight, and leads us to a more accurate understanding of back pain.

In the process of fixing tough cases, variously diagnosed as a disc, arthritis, spinal stenosis, a spondylo, a bone spur, etc., we get the entire purpose of orthopedic-neurological exam – to recreate the familiar pain the patient has been suffering. To hear the patient say *That's it, that's my problem.*

DISC SHMISC

Every time I fix a "disc" case, the patient says, *That's it, that's my problem*, and it's nowhere near a disc. *That's it* is always in the muscles.

You might not get that on the first day, often all they feel in the beginning is pain and soreness. But down the road, as tissues heal, instead of pain, they feel what we're working on and why. They feel where they're at and where they're going, as they feel the exact source of their pain being erased from their body. This is a historic moment in spine medicine.

Before I go into the principles of AMR, let's first take a look at current treatments for back pain.

Treatments

Fix enough of those tough chronic cases when all else has failed, and it teaches you something. It begs for an accounting - why? This is my best explanation . . .

The period 1300 – 1800 AD is known as "the little ice age." A four degree drop in average global temperature set off a time of volatile climactic change, including "the year of no summer." New York harbor was frozen for over five weeks. The east coast had two feet of snow in June and July. In Europe, thousands of Napoleon's soldiers starved and froze to death during one such severe winter. By one soldier's account, although the horse's skin was frozen, the horse continued to move forward through the bitter cold. A soldier would come along with a knife and slice off a piece of flesh to eat. The horse kept on moving as though nothing had happened – it couldn't feel it.

Often, pain is what stops you from moving. Override the sensation of pain and your muscles would still be able to do the job.

Back pain being self-limiting, anything that helps override pain and numb out spasm will at times feel curative. What you're not aware of is the remnant underlying spasm that is numbed out of your awareness. And when you're in pain, it probably doesn't matter.

Thus the actuality of many treatments: Interfere with your perception of pain, help numb out offending fibers, make some bacon, and hopefully you're one of the 80% for whom pain will fade away in a reasonable amount of time.

Overriding the pain gait

The body has an enormous amount of sensory information coming into the brain. Aside from what we see, hear, and smell, sensors are constantly letting you know the position of your joints, if you're moving, being touched, how hard. If you're hot, cold, wet or dry. The number of pain nerves is minor relative to other sensory nerves and the vast amounts of information they relay to the brain every second. If you overload the sensory input, the brain is distracted from perceiving pain signals – overriding the pain gait.

Treatments

Did you know the primary effect of ice and heat is analgesia, or painkilling? A physical form of aspirin. Overload the nervous system with massive thermal nerve input, and you can't feel the pain. Ice also helps reduce swelling, but often, inflammation is not the problem.

NSAIDs - non-steroidal anti-inflammatory drugs. Painkillers like these help to cover up your perception of pain, but they do nothing to fix the problem. They will tell you it helps with inflammation but often inflammation is not the problem. The downside to these drugs are many. Side effects include: indigestion, diarrhea, stomach pain, ulcers, increased risk of heart attack and stroke.

Muscle relaxers have a drug effect that overrides your perception of pain, and while you may feel looser, make no mistake, they do not recondition muscles. It is this author's opinion they leave your muscles a little more tense when they wear off.

Cortisone. I call it inject and pray. Inject with cortisone and pray to god it works. The pain relief is at times amazing, sometimes the relief is temporary, and other times it does nothing at all.

They limit the number of cortisone injections you can receive in a year to 3-4. Why? Because it breaks down connective tissue. It turns muscle into bacon, and ultimately weakens the joint. While sometimes the body is able to absorb the bacon and compensate, what do you do when cortisone doesn't work? And is this really the treatment of choice? Making bacon out of your muscles is not a good idea, and I question whether it's application in the elderly leads to permanent damage.

They also tell you it reduces inflammation, yet again, so often inflammation is another inaccurate model of pain.

Once upon a time doctors lamented the therapeutic benefits of cocaine. One day, cortisone for musculoskeletal conditions will be seen the same way.

Various injections and surgical implants to block pain or deaden nerves are completely baseless and missing the problem.

Prolotherapy injections are aimed at promoting re-growth of collagen to strengthen ligaments. But ligaments are not the problem.

Treatments

Acupuncture interferes with your perception of pain, and helps numb spasm out of your awareness, but it does not recondition muscle.

Physical Therapy.   The stretching and strengthening aspect of physical therapy is great.   There is definitely a time and place for it.   There are moments you can stretch your way out of pain, and it's great for preventing pain.   But there are moments you can't stretch it out, and moments when strengthening only makes it tighter.   Take a bath towel and wring it along its length.   Now pull on each end.   You can stretch it out some, but it's still twisted.   If you have a towel wrung tight, you want to un-wring the towel first, and this of course is what is being missed.

Stretching and strengthening only partially reconditions muscle.

Electrical muscle stimulation?   Yikes.   Let's take an already over contracted muscle and make it contract some more?   An attempt to wear out the spasm and let go its grip?   It's like trying to pacify a crying baby by slapping it.

Ultrasound, in my opinion, is not much better than a hot bath with a rubber duck when it comes to treating back pain.

DISC SHMISC

Traction is nothing more than forced stretching. They will tell you it creates a negative pressure sucking the disc back in, but the disc is irrelevant, the relief is from stretching your muscles.

Sometimes you can get away with forced stretching, and sometimes it will make people worse as muscles tense to resist, further aggravating the underlying spasm pattern. If I pull on your arm, and someone else pulls on the other, by shear force we may stretch out the elastic components of your flesh, but you'd better believe your muscles will be tensing to resist. I'd stick with regular stretching and get your muscles worked on correctly.

I believe chiropractic adjustments break up adhesions in the wrapping between muscles, which is occasionally amazing.

I had a guy come in pinching in his mid-lower spine, walking but unable to bend and tie his shoes. I did a rather exotic move: muscle testing to find the segment to be adjusted and marking it with a wax pencil, then lying him on his back with a block under that segment and giving a quick tug of the leg. He felt it release and the relief was immediate. He felt good as new, could tie his shoes and was completely surprised. I was too, though acted as though it was no big deal.

Treatments

The problem with adjustments, aside from not being able to fix many conditions, is people becoming *addicted* to the adjustment. Because adjustments do not recondition muscle, large programs of adjusting often leave muscles brittle and unstable. You will often hear of people being afraid to open a car door for fear of *losing the adjustment*. What once gave such relief now gives relief that doesn't last so long. People become addicted to the momentary relief of *the crack*. There are also moments when people are hurt by adjustments.

Deep muscle therapy. We have been under the misguided notion you can beat muscles into submission, that pressure melts spasm like a knife through butter. Why? Because so often you can get away with it.

The popular muscle therapies of the day, whether it's "art" / active release, myofascial release, rolfing, shiatsu, acupressure, deep tissue etc., are what I consider gross and over pressing – and I used to do many of them.

To illustrate the point, let's take a look at the column of muscle running down either side of the spine, the erectors. These are postural muscles that hold us upright.

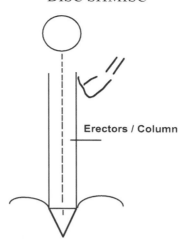

Imagine me, over six foot, over two hundred pounds, leaning on this column with my elbow, and all of my body weight, then moving at a snails pace up or down the column, that's Rolfing - heavy, gross, steamrolling pressure.

Or imagine me just leaning with my elbow, or pressing with a thumb on a tender knot with the instruction, "Just breath, just relax into it," this is acupressure, or deep tissue work.

You may be able to breath and take it, but what you're actually doing is relaxing every other part of your body – you can't help but tense slightly directly under the pressure. It's an autonomic reflex that is beyond your ability to control. Press too heavy or too long on a muscle, and it tenses slightly to resist. By shear force you may break up adhesions between muscles, but layers of muscle are tensing to resist the onslaught.

Treatments

Push on the end of your nose with your thumb using similar pressure. Just breath, just relax. Feel relaxed? I didn't think so. The pressure stimulates sensory nerves overriding the pain gait, distracting you from pain, but muscles tense slightly in response.

Years ago, I had one of those plastic acupressure hooks. One evening the erector in my mid-back was on fire, and applying pressure with the hook gave immediate relief, and allowed me to sleep. Yet the next time I was worked on with AMR, I could tell that some fibers had been clumped together. Until the AMR, I had no clue, it was numbed out of my awareness.

There was a time I thought heavy pressure like this was god's gift to humanity, but the bottom line is – it doesn't work on tough cases, and in some situations will make people worse, as over pressing causes muscles to tense, further aggravating the underlying pattern. Sometimes you notice it right away, other times you notice it a couple days later, you're worse off from the session. I've heard it many times in my career, deep muscle therapy made their condition worse. They don't sue the therapist, they know they had good intention, it only serves to make people think their condition is more serious than it is.

Here's a recent example:

DISC SHMISC

I left a student to care for a difficult case while out of town. We'd been working together on her, making consistent progress after she'd been laid up 7 weeks straight sleeping on the living room floor, life stopped in its tracks; unable to stand, sit or walk, radiating pain and tingling down the leg, her foot numb for days at a time. We were making consistent progress and I encouraged her to continue with my student while away.

Because he was just out of massage school, he didn't yet realize the limitations of what he'd been taught. Instead of continuing as I'd shown, he had to try out some of what he'd learned at school. He thought he was being very gentle, and even she said he was very caring and in constant communication to make sure she was "relaxed", but she had difficulty getting off the table after the treatment, and spiraled down from there as though she were back to square one. When I called to check on her, she was in tears, and inconsolable. What had he done? Just some gentle constant pressure with the thumb, and the instruction "Just breath, just relax."

Resuming with proper treatment, it took a total of one month to get her sitting and driving again, and another month to get her back to work, doing hour-and-a-half sessions once or twice a week. Two doctors had told her she needed surgery for a disc.

Treatments

Gross mashing also lacks refinement. Consider a Ziploc / re-sealable plastic bag. You can mash all over the bag all day long, even along the Ziploc, but you won't open the bag unless you come across the Ziploc at the right angle, at the right location, with your fingers. Very often in the body there are seams or crevices much like the Ziploc on a baggie. You can mash on them all day, and not open them up.

Or consider the sail on a sailboat. On a super windy day, they don't put the sail all the way up, as it's too much power for the boat. So say they put it up half way. All the extra sail at the bottom, they tie it around the boom. If this sail represents a muscle from age, injury, wear and tear, you can massage the sail all day long, it's not going anywhere until you untie it from the boom. Many times in the body, what you think is bone is a boom.

Principles of AMR

With AMR, we do not sit on muscles, or steamroll them, rather we *stroke* them.

Principle 1. The stroke is one-time, and then a complete release of the muscle.

Just as in combing your hair, or raking leaves, *the stroke* is a rhythmic one-time and then a complete release of the muscle. You don't comb your hair back and forth with pressure, and when you rake leaves you pick the rake up between strokes. This is a little thing, and it's everything. Stroke back and forth on a muscle, even with light pressure, and it tenses slightly to resist. This is something you can feel and is easily demonstrated.

There is no constant pressure, no stroking back and forth with pressure, and no dragging. You must release the muscle completely between each stroke. This is huge. You can't fully recondition muscles if they are tensing to resist.

Principle 2. A good stroke has a distinct feel as though strumming your finger across a deck of cards.

I call it playing the body like a one-time deck of cards. The stroke is always one-time, in one direction, and then a complete release of the muscle. We're always looking for angles and locations that give a distinct *deck-of-cards* feeling. When you have it right, both you and the patient will know it.

Notice, to play a guitar you don't sit on the strings. You don't strum a guitar along its strings. You only make that resonant sound if you strum across them.

You don't want to skip across the deck, you want a nice fillet of individual cards. And you want to come across the entire deck, not just half way through. Or, you wouldn't want to separate only a few cards in the middle of the deck, this would be short stroking. Thus, you can fool yourself into thinking you're doing a good stroke, but it's not. Make as long a stroke as possible, strumming as many cards as possible, this will make an enormous difference in the quality / effectiveness of the stroke.

DISC SHMISC

You can't find a deck of cards everywhere. I give students the fundamental map of what I call *universal ins*, a place you can find a deck of cards on anyone - then we try to expand on it. If you lose your way, don't worry, you always have a way *in*. By knowing all the different *ins*, and expanding on them, we connect the dots, and in time you will find good strokes where you could not find them before. Your patient will feel the clumped flesh that is the exact source of their pain.

Looking at muscles in an anatomy book is good for a reference, however, one must remember that this is how they look once dissected. Massive amounts of connective tissue saran wrap removed, to reveal the grain and pattern of muscle. Layers of muscle removed to reveal still deeper layers. We don't have the luxury of working on dissected muscles. We work from the outside-in, from the skin-in.

Also, muscles start out a hot dog and age into bacon. How muscles feel on an 18 year old vs an 80 year old are light years apart, and there's every shade of grey in between. Thus, how muscles look in a book, and how they feel from the outside-in played as a one-time deck of cards are very different things.

Sometimes you are rolling the flesh of a muscle much as it looks in a book. Sometimes you are cleaning out a seam or crevice that you wouldn't know was there. And sometimes you are rolling over what is so often mistaken for bone. Bones don't roll. It is crustified muscular attachment. In each of these situations we are looking for that distinct deck of cards feeling.

I would call this work cross-fiber, but I've taken seminars in cross-fiber, and what they consider cross-fiber and what I consider cross-fiber are worlds apart. They stroke back and forth with pressure – a cardinal sin. They short stroke, miss the crevices and bones, and have no concept of the patterns the way we play them. It's night and day different.

There are two ways to do the stroking:

1. Using oil / lotion.

2. Manipulating skin, or manipulating skin through loose thin clothing. This is more advanced, though there are moments when oil / lotion is a better plan of action.

Doing excellent work does require some hand strength. If your hands are weak, start out using oil / lotion, and with practice you'll develop all the strength necessary to do excellent strokes in either manner. For the record, I have female students five feet tall, and I trust them working on anyone. It's all technique and developing skill with your hands.

Let me give you a couple examples of a universal in.

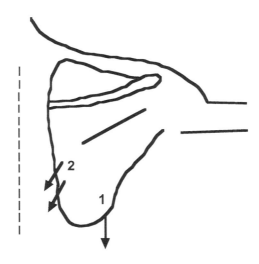

1. Using oil or lotion, use a minimal amount, you want a little bit of traction or feel, as you glide across skin. Using your fingertips like the tines of a leaf rake, you will simply stroke one-time, gliding over skin at the same angle and location as the arrow. Toward the bottom of the scapula, on the side of the rib cage, stroke straight down, there is a very large and distinct deck of cards to be found here rolling flesh. Adjust your location until you find it. You can't follow it very far, find the sweet spot of a good stroke. (I would stand on the left side and reach across.)

2. These arrows represent a universal in on the medial aspect of the shoulder blade. Stroke one time at the same angle and location as the arrows, you will find a smaller deck of cards at the edge of bone and flesh. It will be more pronounced on some, depending on whether they are more hot dog or bacon. Adjust the angle and location until you find it, when you have it right you will know. Follow it as far as you can north or south on the blade, if you lose it, don't worry, you always have a way in. (putting the arm off the front of the table will allow you to follow it north as far as possible.)

See how important angle and location is? Your location can be off a bit and miss it. Your angle can be off and miss it.

Now, compare that with constant, or gross steam rolling pressure, much better, no? If the soil of a garden is hard, you want to till the soil and pluck the fibers apart vs steamrolling and compacting it further.

If you want to try the more advanced manipulating skin method, take the lightest contact with skin in the opposite direction of the arrow, so you can make a longer stroke in the direction of compression – along the arrow. If you don't take skin the other way, you can't stroke very far. You want to move skin all it allows without dragging across it. Make as long a stroke as the skin allows, getting as many cards as possible in the direction of compression.

If you're rowing a boat in a race, you take the oars out of the water and bring them all the way back to make as long a stroke as possible. Same here. Release the entire muscle and bring *skin only* as far back as possible so you can make a longer stroke in the direction of compression.

Rookie mistake #1. You let up off the hard core, but maintain some contact with more superficial layers. You must take your oars out of the water between strokes, just the lightest contact with *skin only* on the way back.

Patients, it's on you to inform them if they aren't letting go of the muscle completely between strokes. It causes just a slight bit of tension and you can take it, but we don't want you to! You must stop them and inform to release completely between strokes. *Skin only*, on the way back. I cannot emphasize this enough.

There's typically a little learning curve to find these strokes, don't be hard on yourself. It's all about angle and location, when you have it right it pops.

You can add more compression so long as your patient is relaxed where you are working. Patients, if there is any doubt, have them lighten up for comparison. The idea is to maximize stimulation so long as completely relaxed where strokes are applied.

That wasn't too bad, no? Now lets go back and look at how we approach the erectors. Depending on who you're working on, these can be a little more challenging.

ERECTORS / COLUMNS

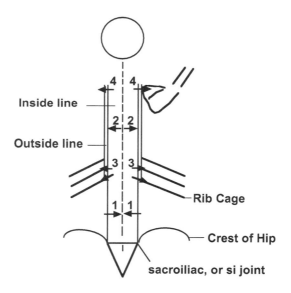

I'll describe the strokes at their most refined, manipulating skin. If using oil / lotion, you may not feel the decks of cards as precisely, but because we don't over press on muscles and are approaching at the correct angle, they will still be very effective.

Principles of AMR

1. Column / Erector at the waist.

The *column at the waist* is one large belly of muscle, ideally stroked in this direction using fingertips. If you go the other way it's not all bad, but there's something important you will miss. In a young person, this *universal in* is easily identified and rolled. For others, it's hard, crusty and difficult to roll. Look for a crevice at the edge of the column, and get as many cards as you can. If you have difficulty, don't worry, we'll cover what to do in a minute.

You can't expand on this *universal in* very far. Often you don't get much more than a way *in*, and do a mantra on the sweet spot of a good stroke. A mantra is focused work on one or several lines for an extended period of time.

Once you hit the crest of the hip, forget it, you're done with this stroke. Same going the other way, once you hit the rib cage, you're done. Most often all you get is a way *in* right at the waist.

From the rib cage to the neck, the erectors split into two entities, the notorious *inside* and *outside* line.

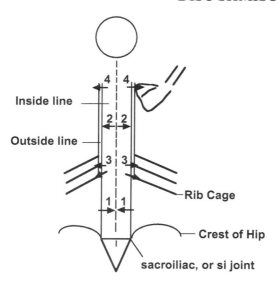

Inside line

Outside line

Rib Cage

Crest of Hip

sacroiliac, or si joint

2. INSIDE LINE

The first roll of muscle away from the boney midline is what I call the *inside line*, and you can follow it a long way. It is a large roll of muscle, it may be fleshy, it may be crusty, depending on who you're working on.

This is always stroked away form midline. Why? Try stroking it the other way and you'll see, the stimulation is not good.

This line is often hard and crusty and you might want to try something other than finger tips:

Edge of hand over thumb – PUSH STROKE

Principles of AMR

I use edge of left hand (as in karate chop), over the back of the right thumb. Middle of right thumb, at joint, is the contact point. Keep the thumb completely relaxed, if you use the thumb you'll kill it. Push with the left hand, or as a unit. Edge of hand over thumb is a PUSH STROKE, pushing away from you.

This offers a little more power which is helpful at times, but be careful, you're still looking for a refined roll of flesh and a deck-of-cards feeling vs a gouge or bounce off the hard core.

Remember, always bring skin back with you to make a longer stroke in the direction of compression, it's not a lot, but it makes all the difference. If you don't take skin the other way, you can't get that many cards, and the stroke is no good.

As you follow it up and down, some hard spots may be acutely sore, while others may be completely numbed out – they can't feel a thing. There's no way you could know what they feel, they are the only ones wired to their body. It can feel hard all along it's path, and parts of it will stick out to the patient as tender, and "Can you tell what I'm feeling?" Honestly, no, it felt just as hard an inch away. This is why your patient is your best guide. We need to get out of this whole notion of thinking we know better than the patient what they feel – you will be mistaken.

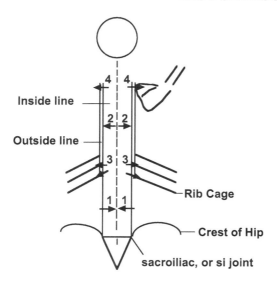

Inside line

Outside line

4 4

2 2

3 3

1 1

Rib Cage

Crest of Hip

sacroiliac, or si joint

3/4 OUTSIDE LINE

After this first big roll of muscle there is a little crevice that is not obvious, and you wouldn't even know it was there. Clean out this crevice, there is a distinct deck of cards to be found here that is very important – the *outside line*.

This *outside line* is a good example of the Ziploc bag, and the specificity of what we are looking for. You can mash on it all day and miss it entirely. Ideally this is a fingertip stroke that gets to the essence of this work – refinement.

3. You can always find a way in stroking down and out on the lower rib cage, then straight out as you follow it up. It might get a little muddled by the blade, don't worry, as you have seen, there's other things we do there.

Bring skin with you across the crevice so you can make a longer stroke back, sinking into the crevice and separating as many cards as possible. If you start your stroke right at the crevice, it's a short stroke and not good.

This is the art and science of it. As in martial arts, there are white, green, blue and black belts, though because we don't over press on muscles, even average strokes can be very effective treating serious back pain.

Just right pressure: it requires varying degrees of hand strength to unravel this crevice. You can press too hard looking for it and miss it. You can use too little pressure to delineate.

Again, use all that the skin gives you and get as many cards as possible. Your patient will notice a large difference in the quality / effectiveness of the stroke. And now you see why I started you out on the shoulder blade. For the beginner, doing excellent strokes here takes a little practice. If using oil, you will simply start on the inside line, and let your fingers sink into the crevice as you stroke away from midline. It won't be as specific as manipulating skin, but because we aren't over pressing, and are approaching at the proper angle, it will still be effective.

4 There is another *universal in* stroking straight away right over the top of the blade, right over skin and bone.   (arm off the front of the table is often helpful, or off to side works on many)

As you work these lines, your client will tell you which line is on fire. It may be the *inside line*, the *outside line*, or both. It could vary as you go up and down the spine.

Working the *inside* and *outside line* in this manner will spoil you from typical deep muscle therapies.

Let me give you a little more perspective on spasm patterns.

SPASM PATTERNS SPREAD

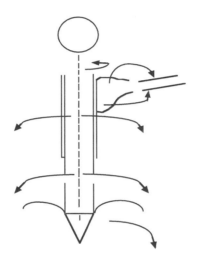

If we're standing in a crowded room and I'm a little tipsy, I'm going to hang onto you for support. If you're tipsy, you're going to hang onto the person next to you for support. And this is what happens with muscle fibers, they cling to the one next for support.

As we age, spasm patterns spread. What was once a hard core in an otherwise fleshy muscle, now involves the whole muscle, which feels hard as a rock.

Where once knots and ropes used to accumulate in muscles individually, now groups of muscles are clumping and shrink wrapping together. The erector / column in the low back starts reaching around the waist and into the abdomen and groin for support. In the mid-back they reach further out into the rib cage for help. Below the waist, they shrink wrap around the hip, and like a towel wrung tight start descending and involving more and more of the leg.

FROM THE LIVING TO THE DEAD

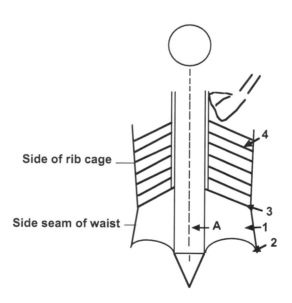

For many, the *column at the waist*, and the *outside line* is a good place to start, and you need not go wider. But, if these are insensitive, or numbed out, and good strokes there don't feel like they're doing anything, they may wake up with a bit of work, or it may be helpful to go wider. As you go wider, there is always an easy way *in* that with finger tip pressure you can find tissue that is alive, sensitive, and a refined stroke that feels like it's doing something.

Then when you come back to the columns that were numbed out, they are more alive and receptive to treatment. I call this working from the outside-in, or from living to the dead

A Column at the waist

A represents the *column at the waist*, as previously described. For some, the column will be *it*, and going any wider they'll say, *what are you doing* ?

1 Side seam of the waist

For others, the column will be hard as a rock, numb / insensitive, and difficult to roll. There is always a deck of cards next to the one you're working on. Explore laterally, you'll start to find some cards, but keep going and find the sweet spot of the next deck of cards, what I call the *side seam of the waist*. For some, you may have to go all the way around to the abdomen to find this. For many, both the *column*, and the *side seam* will feel involved.

2 ASIS (front / side of crest)

Muscles reef on here like the sail on a sail boat. An important universal *in* you can find a on anyone, rolling flesh over bone. It can get real bunched up here requiring a mantra.

(patient lying on side may be an easier position to get these)

3 Lowest boney edge of rib cage.

Angle up on the lowest boney edge of the rib cage. This becomes another reefed sail, and very important. This will feel like nothing more than skin and bone - and a deck of cards.

This is typically more sensitive, and you will have to adjust your stroke lighter going over the ribs. You can then follow this higher up the rib cage. Start your stroke wide, on the side of the rib cage, wiggle skin and see where it lets you into a deck of cards right over the ribs and follow it back as far as possible.

4 Fibers cross-stitch on the rib cage, as you come up, you can also angle down.

For the beginner, this is how easy we can make it.

ERECTORS MADE EASY

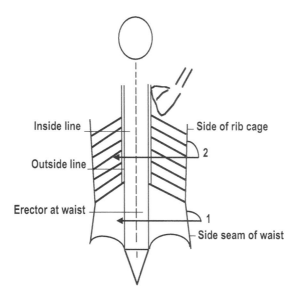

Inside line — Side of rib cage

2

Outside line —

Erector at waist —

1

Side seam of waist

1 Side seam / Column at waist

This arrow represents a long stroke using oil. Reach around the abdomen, all the way to the belly button if you like, set you're your fingers like the tines of a leaf rake and do a long stroke all the way back.

Look for a deck of cards at the *side seam of the waist*, and at the *column at the waist*. Finish strong all the way over the midline, as for some this is involved.

I often put one hand over the other for support to maximize stimulation.

Of course you can angle up on the rib cage, and down on the crest of hip as shown previously.

2 Rib cage / Inside / Outside line

Reach around the *side of the rib cage* and stroke back across, don't stop early, finish strong over the *inside / outside line* on the opposite side.

You are treating accurately the *rib cage* on the right, and the *inside / outside line* on the left.

Just doing these two strokes alone will produce amazing results for the masses.

We are stroking one time and releasing the muscle. We are approaching fibers at the angle of de-clumping.

THE BIG PICTURE OF SPASM PATTERNS

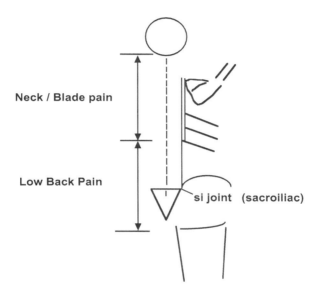

When someone comes in with any neck or mid-back complaint, I'm thinking of a pattern between the base of the skull and the lower rib cage at minimum, not just the spot that hurts.

Someone may come in with pain that localizes in the neck, yet as we work the bigger picture of the pattern, we'll hit areas coming off the blade and they'll say, *That's it! Wow, I had no idea that was part of it.* So we always think of a bigger pattern than just the spot that hurts.

For the low back, I'm thinking lower rib cage to the lower glutes, (butt muscles) – at minimum.   For radiating pain and nerve symptoms down the leg, I'm simply thinking of patterns down the leg.

In the low back, I've had patients whose perception of pain was straight across the low back (L5-S1), yet as we worked the bigger picture of the pattern, the live line, where the patient said, *that's it,* was way down in the lower glute (butt muscle) on one side.

Let me share with you now the classic low back pattern.

1. OPEN UP THE WAIST

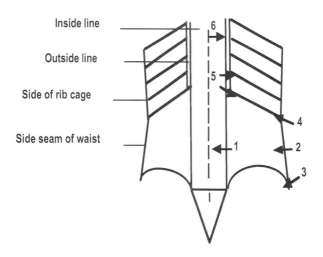

You have already been introduced to one half of the low back pattern. I call this portion *opening up the waist*.

1. Column / Erector at the waist

2. Side seam of the waist

3. Front / side of crest (ASIS)

4. Lower rib cage

5/6. Inside and outside line of the column.

Follow the column up as far as it feels involved.

Muscles can tweak anywhere, any one of these lines may be the *it* line, and they may all feel involved.

Because it's all connected, just as one freeway leads to another, releasing tension in the neck and blade can help low back pain.

2. AROUND THE HORN

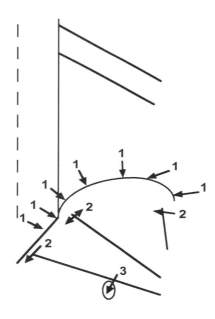

1. Around the Horn – NORTH

This is a major example of the reefed sail and what the whole world is missing, stroking right over what you think is skin and bone.

From the left, this is the start of going *around the horn* from the *north* side of the crest – a *universal in* you must know. It's between midline and the lower inside edge of the si joint.

This is a refined finger tip stroke on a micro deck of cards. Move the skin in either direction all that it gives you and get as many cards as possible. It's not that many, but it makes a big difference

From the right, this is the front / side of the crest (ASIS) as described above under *opening up the waist* – another *universal in* you must know.

Ideally, you would be able follow it all the way around getting a precise deck of cards. Surely there is a way *in* at each end, then try to connect the dots. For some you might have it, lose it, then find it again. In time you will find good strokes where you could not find them before.

As you go *around the horn – north*, it is easy to slip over onto the south side. I want to make you very aware, there is a very important line on NORTH side of the crest. Some people have a pie crust on the crest of their hip, and to stay on the north side you are much higher on the waist than you would expect. At times this whole line is the *it* line. Other times *it* will localize to a portion around the si joint, your patient will tell you, as often there is no way you could know.

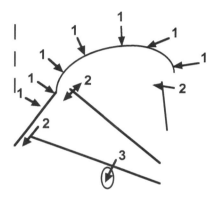

2. Around the horn – SOUTH

From the left, the first 2 is a large deck of cards, an easy *universal in* you can find on anyone going right along the lower boney edge of the sacrum. Finger tip, or push stroke works well here, and as usual, for some this could be *it*.

Around the horn – south begins at the edge of bone, but as you go around you'll be more in the flesh. As you follow around the horn from the south side, get whatever deck of cards you can, you should find some major rolls at the other #2's (glute med / min). It may be beneficial to put them on their side, or a position in between face down and side, to get the lateral ones depending on who you're working on.

These are the glutes / butt muscles which then attach to the femur at the hip. On some you can follow these muscles from one attachment to the other much as it looks in a book. For most you can't. Take what the body gives you, and work the decks at each attachment

3. Butt bone

This is not part of *around the horn*, but it is an important *universal in* you must know and can find on anyone. It feels like a crevice and is rolled right over the butt bone. Push or pull stroke depending on who you're working on, and side position is often helpful to get this.

3. GLUTES / butt muscles

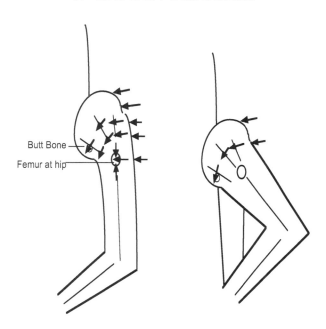

Butt Bone
Femur at hip

You may want to try the side position to work the butt muscles, or perhaps a position in between stomach and side with one knee up. Never be afraid to play with positioning and see what works best for each part of the pattern you're working. Depending on who you're working on these glute seams can take a little oomph to clean out. A push stroke works well here, and if there was ever a place to use the elbow, the meat of the butt muscles would be it.

Just remember to release the muscle completely – pick that rake up between strokes. Refinement is preferred, but not everyone has the strength to make a refined stroke with fingertips. Muscles shrink wrap around the hip socket, and that boney prominence of the *femur at hip* is a place where more than one angle will work. Again, it feels like nothing more than skin and bone, but when you find a deck of cards there, your patient will say, "Thank you, thank you, thank you." There are some extra arrows there. There's always a deck of cards next to the one you're working on.

4. MIDLINE

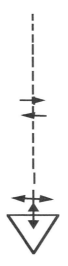

DISC SHMISC

These dashes represent the boney bumps down the midline of your spine, or spinous processes.

For many there is not much to find here, but in the low back and mid-back, you can usually find a deck of cards stroking right over what you think is skin and bone.

Others have a crusty line that runs the entire length of their spine, and will sing your praises for treatment along its length.

Often this line is not involved, but when it is, it can be the center of their universe, and you will have to do a mantra on a deck of cards that what would appear to be nothing but skin and bone. When the tweak is dead center of the lower spine, you'll feel the same deck of cards you would feel if they weren't in pain. There is no way you could know by feeling that it was the core of their condition, they'll tell you. If this is the *it* line, I will change positions and have them bend over the table, or get on their knees on top of the table to expose fibers hiding from treatment in the arch of the low back. There will be one little spot your patient will want you to do a mantra on. In the low back, this is an area you can go two directions and get a deck of cards

CLASSIC LOW BACK PATTERN

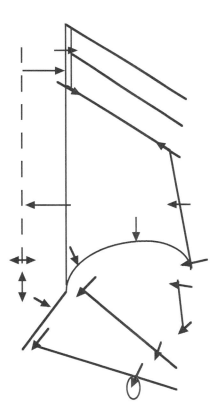

(shown on one side to avoid arrow overload)

Taken together then, this is the classic low back pattern. For many – this is it. For others, the pattern has spread and you'll have to work further around, into the abdomen / groin, or down the leg to resolve.

As you investigate these lines you will discover what's involved and what's not – just ask your patient, often there is no way you could know. For example, one week I had three people come in, their perception of pain identical - straight across the low back. Yet for one person, the *it* line was the *column at the waist*, for another, *it* was *around the horn-north*, and for another, *it* was the *butt bone* on one side. Most of the time, the only thing I can tell is that I have what feels like a decent stroke, there's no way I could know it was their *it* line.

I've also had patients whose pain located to the low back on one side, yet the key to fixing them was working further around into the abdomen / groin. People and conditions come in every shade of grey. Each case is a puzzle to solve. I give you tools to figure each person out.

You don't have to work each side equally. Often only one side will feel involved. Or one side is majorly involved, and the other side is minorly involved. (and occasionally the tweak is dead center)

Principles of AMR

More than anything, go by feel. When the minor side wants some attention, it will talk to you.

Here's my favorite test:

Say you've been working parts of the pattern for a bit and you're not sure where to go or what to do next. Have your client get off the table, walk around and feel it out. Ask them for feedback. Most often their body will talk to them, and they'll tell you what part wants more attention. Sometimes it's, "keep working right where you were," other times, "it wants some attention over here now." If they can't give you any feedback, keep working the most "live", or tender, lines.

It's also a good idea to do this test 10 minutes before the end of a session as things can shift.

Case in point: I was young with juicy muscles the first time my low back went out doing the most simple movement. I went straight to the ground and was stuck there, sharp jabbing nerve pain that felt as though, indeed, a disc was pinching a nerve. It was frightening and felt deadly serious, I couldn't imagine ever being able to walk normally again.

DISC SHMISC

It felt as though I had a 2x4 piece of lumber next to my spine, and I had that classic look that anyone who's been through it can empathize: hobbling, tilted over, looks like you got hit in the butt with a shovel, grimacing as deep jolts of nerve pain pierced the si joint. It feels like anything but a muscle.

Fortunately, my girlfriend, who was an expert and introduced me to this work, assured me not to worry. As she worked the entire pattern I could feel how all the muscles were involved, primarily on the left side. As it melted it came down to one last core, the source of my pain, the attachments to the left si joint. (around the horn - north, left side.) She put me in touch with the exact source of my problem and it surprised the heck out of me.

* * *

I say one side of your back is major, and the other side is minor. Balance is a nice idea, but our bodies don't have it. Just as one side of your face looks different from the other, the state of your muscles differs from one side to the other, and it goes beyond handedness, to our constitution.

I'm right handed, yet the entire left side of my body has a more advanced spasm pattern. For other right hander's it's just the opposite. Yes, overuse can certainly come into play, but often it defies logic.

For me it was the left si joint, and the left mid-back that were always symptomatic, and wanting attention. Stroking there felt tender and provided relief to the source of my pain. Stroking the right felt normal, no tenderness, and it didn't feel involved.

As we age, patterns spread and reach across the spine into the "good" side. In the beginning it was always the left side that was the symptomatic, or major side. Now I can have pain on the right. The underlying pattern is still worse on the left, but either side can tweak, and when it does, that's it - it doesn't matter that the overall pattern is worse on the left, the right side wants more attention.

The left side, which was once the more tender side, has turned into bacon, can't feel it even when stroked. Now the right side feels more tenderness to the touch, not because it's better, only because it's more alive than the dead / bacon side.

Also, while that first time there was that 2x4 knot of spasm sticking out next to the spine, in later episodes nothing stuck out, there was no apparent spasm. Thus the understandable position we find ourselves in today: diagnosing based on how it feels (like a nerve), and what we see on x-ray or MRI (a disc or a joint).

I don't want to bore you with how we treat the entire body here, it's not the purpose of the book. It's meant to give you an example of the very tangible differences in how we approach muscles / back pain. There are many muscle therapies that have the same intention, and sound similar in words: it's meant to recondition muscles, it feels deep etc., but as you can see, there's a big difference between gross mashing and precision raking.

Learning to do the work

I remember only too well how lost I was when first converting to this work despite all previous training, and having it done on my own body. When I was worked on by an expert, the strokes were made with exacting precision. I remember clearly how lost I felt when attempting to reproduce those strokes on my own.

There is a bit of a learning curve. For me, having it done on my own body, I didn't have a choice but to stick with it and treat others the way I wanted to be treated myself. As with many things, practice makes perfect, and in time it will all become clear. You make what we call step changes, something clicks and your hands just became a little smarter. This will happen for weeks, months and years down the road.

In time what you're looking for in a good stroke will become second nature. Once you have the fundamentals down, you won't have to think about what you're doing, your hands will go on autopilot, searching and destroying underlying spasm, flowing from one good stroke to another with artful precision.

If you practice, what you observe will never cease to amaze you. You will gain newfound confidence in your ability to not only give relief, but actually fix things.

Inflammation

Inflammation is another inaccurate model of pain, at least most of the time. I can't tell you how many times someone has come in diagnosed with a disc, causing inflammation and putting pressure on a nerve. If they were truly inflamed I should be making them worse. So how is it they get off my table with less pain, and better motion? Obviously inflammation was not the problem.

Inflammation, like so many diagnoses, is just another catch-all phrase. If you're in pain, something must be inflamed, or you wouldn't be in pain.

For a sprained ankle, inflammation is obvious and you don't work on the puffy swelling. In the spine however, and in so many conditions, inflammation is simply an inaccurate model of pain, and is not the problem. How to tell? It can be difficult. If something is swollen stay off it.

If you're not sure, do this test: work very lightly for a few minutes with their permission, then get them up off the table and see how they react. Taking guarding spasm away from a truly inflamed joint will make them less stable, the joint is not ready to handle the extra motion, and they'll know it as soon as they stand up. If they are less stable, you'll have to let the swelling settle down a couple days before going to work on it. If they are no worse, or slightly better, you can continue to work. If you still aren't sure, work a few more minutes and test it out again.

In 25 years of admittedly low volume work, there has only been a handful of times I could not go directly to work on an acute back / neck.

If they are inflamed you can work around the inflammation, often to great effect. In the sprained ankle for example, we don't work on the swelling, but the shock of the injury sets off a reactive spasm in the entire muscle, which runs all the way up to the knee. Working way up in the calf, away from the swelling, starts taking the muscles out of shock / reactive spasm.

When you sprain a ligament, you have damaged muscle as well, and it is the reactive spasm from injury that never gets reconditioned properly.

Example. Karen, a woman in her 40's comes in. She'd been to not one, but four, "famous" orthopedists from across the country. The best diagnosis they could come up with was "bursitis" of the hip, or inflammation of a fluid filled sac surrounding the hip joint. She'd been on anti-inflammatories for the better part of a year. Physical therapy had helped some, but a year later she was still in a lot of pain, and unable to cross her legs. If you could watch me work, if she was indeed inflamed, I should be making her worse. Yet, each time she got off the table she felt better. Five one-hour sessions later she comes in, "Brian, I can't believe it, I can cross my legs again, I'm almost completely well, I can't believe it!"

The course of treatment

People and conditions come in every shade of grey. The vast majority will notice some improvement right away. Any improvement after the first session is a good sign, even if it doesn't last, as for extreme cases it can take a number of sessions just to make a dent.

For a bad low back, what you notice first is less pain and better motion around the core of your condition, but the core remains. Treatments give relief but it doesn't last, and "the grip" of spasm starts setting back in.

Think of your spasm pattern as the cross section of a tree trunk. Each time we work we'll take a couple rings off the outside. As you lie on the table, there is no stress going through the muscles, and because we stroke them just right, even the trunk that remains will relax a bit. But once you go back to standing / sitting and putting stress through the trunk, it is very easy to aggravate, and when you do, it can feel like you're back to square one. You aren't back to square one, the rings we took off are still missing, it's the trunk that remains that got set off.

With each treatment we take off more and more rings, treatments last longer and longer until it's all just a bad memory. You find yourself doing things without thinking about it, and it hits you, you remember this was something you couldn't do not that long ago.

As you come out of it, it is common for the pain to move around. It might localize to a place you hadn't felt before. As pain dies down in one area, other areas are being heard. They're all part of the pattern. We just keep putting out fires until they're all gone.

It's not always a straight line to success, especially for chronic conditions. It is common that as you are able to do more, you aggravate it from lifting, or over doing it. Again, you haven't lost all we have gained, rather aggravated the trunk that remains. We just to treat it, and go forward. If you want to test / push your ability, do it right before a treatment in case you aggravate something.

For a bad low back, our job is to recondition your pattern, your job is the following:

1. Walk.

For a bad low back walking is not an option, you must walk. Walking is the #1 exercise you can do for a bad low back. 30 minutes twice a day would be nice.

First and foremost, listen to your body and do what's right in the moment. When locked up in acute pain, perhaps half a block is all you can do. Down the road you may find tremendous benefit from an hour walk.

2. Wag your tail.

When your low back goes out, you will notice it involves the muscles that would wag your tail if you had one. While lying around, wag your tail: forward, backward, and side to side. Don't force it through the core that is stuck, but try to move around it in all directions.

For other areas of the body, work to regain your normal range of motion, again, without forcing through something that feels stuck. Work around what the body gives you.

3. Avoid sitting.

Sitting is the most stressful position on the spine. If you have a bad low back, sitting will bring it out. If you must sit, a ball is much better than a chair as it will diffuse forces going through the pattern. Take frequent breaks to walk and stretch.

4. Stretch

Stretching and strengthening is the perfect compliment to this work, but getting your muscles reconditioned in this manner is the primary component that is currently being missed.

When coming out of acute or chronic injury I believe fluid motion stretching is safer – just as it sounds, moving fluidly into and out of a stretch. While there are times you can get away with forceful stretching, fluid motion is safer.

In general you want to re-establish pain free range of motion before adding resistance exercises.

DISC SHMISC
If your back is on edge of going out

If you get into trouble and feel your back about to go out, do the following:

A. Walk. Sometimes you can walk yourself right out of an episode.

B. Biopulser. If you have a biopulser*, use it. It has happened to me that I was getting out of bed and my back started going out, right into splinting spasm. I fell back into bed, reached for the bio-pulser and prevented the event.

C. Lie on your back. Put your feet up on a chair or something so that your knees are over your hips. (as if you were sitting in a chair, only lying on your back) Lie there, read a book, watch tv. Breathe, drawing your navel to your spine. Lie like this for long periods, and aside from that, walk.

D. AMR. The best thing is to get this treatment. Often you will have a warning sign your back is on the verge of going out. Listen to your intuition and prevent it.

* The biopulser is Griner's invention, sort of a jackhammer for the body that helps break up underlying spasm. (see biopulser.com) A quick percussive blow stimulates the hard core of the spasm without making it tense. Again, everything we do is an attempt to stimulate muscles without making them tense.

The biopulser is a great helper, offering real benefit, but it does not replace the hand work. There is something the hands do the biopulser does not. It is a great combination however.

Many massagers on the market that vibrate and go bzzzz are too fast. The vibration distracts from pain, but muscles actually tense slightly in response - worthless in my opinion. Then there are the slow roller / kneading type massage devices. Like typical massage, too slow, heavy, and unrefined.

The biopulser is the only machine I recommend at the moment, and I make nothing for saying that – no stock, no money, no travel, no dinner, no biopulsers, no nothing.

Questions that remain

For all I can tell you about back pain, patients do not like me for what I can't tell them - the inevitable questions.

How much treatment will it take to fix your conditon?

How long should treatment sessions be?

When should I be treated again?

How much treatment will it take to fix your condition?

To this day, this is the most difficult question to answer – I never know. Occasionally I can venture a guess, but most often, *I don't know, it takes what it takes*, is my honest answer. And that's the horrible truth people do not like to hear. Sure, for the masses 1-10 weekly hour or half-hour sessions will suffice, but how can you tell if they'll fall into the category masses? You can't. You never know who will turn into a tough chronic case and who will not.

Example A. *Saul, 20's, was helping to unload a heavy piece of equipment. He didn't notice anything at the moment, but the next morning he couldn't get out of bed, acute low back pain, radiating nerve pain down the leg. He went to the emergency room, they take an MRI, there's no disc. They say, "Here, take some pain medications, you'll be fine." For the masses, they will be. But in his case, a year-and-a-half of medication, physical therapy, and chiropractic and he was still disabled.*

Example B. *Brad, 30's, had felt tight and sore from playing a lot of tennis, no big deal he thought, until his back went out, excruciating pain radiating to the foot. They take an MRI, there's no disc to blame it on.*

He tried cortisone, both oral and injected, several chiropractors, physical therapy, and different types of deep muscle therapy, which sometimes gave temporary relief, and sometimes made him worse. All in all, he couldn't walk well for six months, and was in chronic pain for a year after that when he found his way in.

There you go, no disc on MRI, young fleshy muscles, yet they developed chronic conditions. When I feel their muscles, they feel better than mine. Yet theirs are symptomatic, mine aren't. My bacon is holding stable. It's Einstein's theory of relativity applied to muscles. Relative to how they were before the injury, the reactive contraction has their muscles wrung tight like a washcloth, and never been treated correctly. Relative to mine, they feel fleshy, and I would have no idea they were symptomatic. When they come to see me having been disabled for a year and a half, how could I know if they could be fixed in ten sessions? If they came to me to begin with how could I know? Most often there's no way you could know. Each case, it takes what it takes.

Conversely, you can have degenerated patterns that are holding stable. Or degenerated patterns that are symptomatic, yet resolve quickly. You never know. It surprises me how little it takes. It surprises me how much it takes. The bottom line is how you feel. When you're fixed you will feel it, you won't have to think about it. Here are a few examples to illustrate the gamut.

Example 1   low back - short

I was leaving a store one day, when I see a woman folded over the counter, her toes not touching the ground. It didn't look right and I asked if she was ok. She said that upon getting out of the car, her back went out. She got to the counter and was now stuck there wondering what to do, she had many plans for the evening. I introduced myself and told her that while she may not know me, her condition happened to be my specialty. I start to work the right sacroiliac attachments while she rested, folded over the counter. (around the horn – north)

After several minutes I start thinking to myself, "What are you doing? It takes what it takes to fix these things. There's no guarantee you're going to do anything for her in a few minutes. She could be no better, and sore from the treatment, she's going to think you're a nut." But, we got lucky. After 15 minutes we tested it, and it was gone. She was able to stand, walk, and made all her scheduled engagements. She was surprised and so was I. (note: if inflammation was the problem, I should have made her worse, obviously inflammation was not the problem.)

Example 2   low back - long

When John's low back went out, it was diagnosed as a herniated disc and he suffered chronic low back pain for about two years. It was affecting every aspect of life. He felt like an old man getting out of bed. Couldn't pick up his kids, or chase them down the hall. He estimated about ten injections of cortisone and was just about to undergo surgery when he was referred in as a last resort. He felt enough relief after one session to give me a chance.

It wasn't a straight line to success. As he felt better and tried to do more, he would have an acute flare up from lifting a case of wine or a large piece of art. He would come in gimping, and would be amazed that in one session he could get off the table with no pinch, right back to where we'd left off. It took the better part of a year doing weekly hour to hour-and-a-half sessions to fix him, and as usual he came to understand what his "disc" condition was really all about.

Example 3   neck – short

Stan woke up one morning with pain in his neck. He had no idea what caused it, the only thing he could think of was that he had been lying on a lounge chair looking down to read the day before.

While he went to the office, the pain kept getting progressively worse, so he got a referral to a chiropractor. After the chiropractor he went back to the office, but the pain continued to get worse. "By the time I got home it had frozen up on me. It hurt every time I tried to swallow." His wife called an orthopedist who said to take aspirin and stay in bed. The next morning he couldn't move his neck an inch, and his wife got a referral to me.

On arrival his neck was locked and frozen, he used his feet to turn his torso to look around. I worked on him for an hour and a half, and . . . "That night I went to a cocktail party." (note: if inflammation was the problem, I would have made him worse, obviously inflammation was not the problem.)

Example 4   neck - long

Ted was in his early 30's, loved nature, mountain climbing and skiing. He'd done a lot of traveling and experienced many forms of bodywork. Years earlier while in Los Angeles he was referred in for some minor problem and developed a great appreciation for the work.

Years later he was enrolled in a course to become a certified ski guide. He had injured his neck prior to taking the course but didn't want to cancel. It would be stiff in the morning, loosen up some during the day, and then stiffen up at night. The last day of class they were taught how to carry people down the mountain. At the end he was in bad shape and drove straight to LA from Colorado thinking I'm the man can fix him.

When he got here his neck was also locked and frozen, using his feet to turn his torso to look around. He couldn't even lie down, and slept sitting on a couch with pillows under his arms. Normally, inflammation is not the problem, but in Ted's case, you could brush a feather across the back of his neck and he would scream bloody murder. Inflammation was a problem. So you work around it, normally to some benefit.

Six one-hour sessions with Ted and we hadn't made a dent, at which point he freaked, got an MRI which showed a disc and started seeking all manner of therapies. He was told, "You'll never ski or climb again." A chiropractor adjusted him, made him worse, now he had numbness and tingling radiating into his right hand. At this point I had a little moxie from fixing tough cases and

119

told him, "I think I can fix you, I just think it's going to take some time."

After experimenting with other therapies, he realized it was going to be me or surgery. He stopped the other treatments and we went to hour-and-a-half sessions twice a week on his right neck and blade pattern alone.

It took 8.5 months to fix him, and, as usual, he came to feel the exact nature of his condition – a deeply gripping neck and blade pattern. His shoulder blade was sucked into his spine and when it finally released it dropped a full inch or two away. He's called the last several winters from the ski slopes to thank me.

How long should sessions be?

If I want to fix a tough case and not fail, the only way I can be sure is to not put a time limit on it, and work until I know we've given it a good *what for*, and we both agree, *that's enough for today*.

It's different for everyone, that could be anywhere from 30 minutes to typically, 1.5 – 2 hour sessions. I have a stroke case, partially paralyzed right side, he can get around very slowly with a cane, and often requires a wheel chair. To work on him in this manner, it's a three hour session. We did this once to see what it took, but do we get to work like this? No. Who can afford it? I work on him every month or two to keep his neck out of pain. But if he were able to get regular treatments like this, who knows what is possible?

More than one client in debilitating pain has commented over the years that longer sessions are exponentially better. And I agree, there is no substitute for time. But is this always necessary? No. For the masses, regular hour sessions will suffice, and for many you can get away with less. How can you tell who needs what? I don't know.

3. When should you be treated again?

Ideally? Whenever you're ready for another. Here's my favorite case to illustrate the point. I once made a house call to Hawaii. Marshall's back had gone out on him and they were concerned about him being able to get on a plane at the end of vacation, much less get back to work.

When I arrived late in the afternoon he was in bad shape, unable to stand or walk. He lay there like a turtle on its back, unable to turn over, sharp jolts of pain piercing the left sacroiliac joint.

I worked several hours on him that night and made him gimp for half a block afterward, he, tilted over to one side, looking like he got hit in the butt with a shovel.

DISC SHMISC

The next day he was still hobbling and had a belt line of bruising across his low back from me working on him. That night we drugged him up and worked right through the bruises for several more hours.

The next day he was walking decently, and it was the optimism of an avid golfer that said, "This golf course, Princeville, is amazing, you've got to play it. I'll treat if you can get me swinging before you leave."

We made a tee time for the next day, would work hard on it that night and determine in the morning whether he could swing a club. That day I made him do all manner of exercises wherein he would aggravate something and it would start to pinch. I'd rub it out with a few strokes and make him resume exercises.

That night I went into a zone working and listening to music, our mantra, "We want to play golf in the morning." The next thing you know the sun is rising and the birds are chirping, yikes, I'd worked right through the night, about 6-7 hours, better get some sleep.

We wake up late and are now running late for the tee time. The story behind the story that makes it such a classic is this: Marshall's father was an avid golfer. One morning a foursome is missing one and his father is invited to join at the last minute. He rushes out to the first tee, no warm up, and when he goes to hit the ball his back goes out. He was never able to play golf again in his life due to his bad back. Now we're rushing to the course and we don't know if Marshall can swing a club yet.

We're on the first tee taking some practice swings, he's swinging nice and easy, and I say, "Marshall, if you swing like that we've got no problems."

Marshall tees his ball and this being the island of Kauai, a micro mini rain cloud is overhead raining only on him. I'm standing off the tee dry as a bone. You can't write this stuff. I say, "Marshall, this must be some kind of moment of truth for you buddy."

When he goes to hit the ball he tries to kill it and goes rolling to the ground. "Marshaaall! Are you ok?" "Yeah, I'm fine. I tried to kill it and thought I'd better roll defensively."

He was ok and we played 18 holes of golf. That night we sat in a restaurant with his wife and kids. To anyone who has suffered an acute episode like that, you know, those are two things you wouldn't even consider.

Two conclusions:
1. If inflammation was the problem, I should have been making him worse. Obviously, inflammation was not the problem.

2. This case is my default answer when people ask when they should be treated again - there are no laws. Some people can take this, others want time to heal up between sessions. It's all up to you. We adjust everything to the individual.

Aside from this acute episode, the larger story of Marshall is, he was another who suffered chronic pain for several years that affected every aspect of life. He sought treatment from a variety of doctors and chiropractors all over the world, traveling as a location scout. It took a little over a year of weekly hour to hour-and-a-half sessions to resolve his chronic low back condition.

"This treatment is unlike anything else out there. It has changed my life. The other treatments felt like maintenance, where your work feels curative. It's the only work that I've ever experienced that cures you as opposed to just relief. I remember when you said to get whatever kind of car you want, I thought you were nuts. I had lived with it so long, it had become part of the decision making process."

That was about ten years ago. Recently he had this to say, "Probably the greatest testament to your work is that I really haven't done any of the stretching or exercise you recommended and I'm still stable."

Drawbacks to AMR

AMR is a beautiful thing, the only drawback is that it's work, the sort that makes most people run, not walk, the opposite direction. And while you can mail it in and do very well for the masses, to prove my point, you will have to develop some skill, do extended sessions and give it your all.

With AMR, each stroke is like the swing of a golf club, performed with varying levels of skill and effectiveness. If you want to prove AMR wrong, it will be easy - failures are discussed in the appendix. If Tiger Woods lets me swing the club for him, it's unlikely he will make the cut in a PGA tournament. But it will be proven right, over and over, by those giving souls who develop some skill and do the work.

Fixing tough cases can be like rowing a boat across the ocean. There will be moments when you will question what you're doing, "Am I kidding myself? Will this ever change?" Yes, it will, if you keep working and following the guidelines. Having done it many times, I know what is possible, but I never said it was easy. You will earn your results, and when you do, you get the big understanding. There is no better way to learn and own this work than to fix a tough case. Take someone in chronic pain, been let down by all manner of therapy and take them to the promise land. Do that a few times and you own it . . .

Summation

A doctor once wrote that on the first day of medical school, they were told that fully half of what they were about to learn would turn out to be wrong in the end, they just didn't know which half it would be. It turns out at least a portion of it is the part concerning back pain.

The seeming logical idea of a disc pinching a nerve has not held up to scrutiny. The truth is, when it comes to back pain, the hard evidence makes no sense. Let me emphasize the facts regarding discs one more time as, at the moment, the public remains thoroughly conditioned on the idea of a disc pinching a nerve.

- The disc can herniated to the right, looks like it's pinching the nerve root going down the right leg, but the pain goes down the left leg.

Summation

- Discs routinely shrink or disappear on subsequent MRI all on their own, yet symptoms remain.

- There are people that have no disc on MRI, yet they have chronic radiating nerve pain to the foot.

- There are people with herniated discs, yet they've never had a back pain in their life.

- It's not a question, it's a conclusion in medical literature, there is no correlation between discs and back pain.

Within the industry it's common knowledge – half the population over age forty have a disc, arthritis, stenosis, something deemed significant on x-ray or MRI, yet they have no symptoms. If you have one of these defects and are not in pain, it's said to be asymptomatic, or not causing symptoms. But if you are suddenly in pain, they'll take a picture and blame whatever they see. What else could it be?

It is only too understandable why we have been stuck on these outdated models. The symptoms feel nothing like a muscle, there's no apparent spasm, and what can you say when pain becomes chronic and fails to resolve with all manner of conservative and muscle therapy?

DISC SHMISC

As a chiropractor, I too was frustrated treating chronic back pain – I couldn't fix chronic pain cases, and deferred to orthopedists as the experts.

The confusing aspect of back pain is that so many treatments work at times. For 80% of the population in pain, it doesn't matter who they see, or what treatment they get, it all works. There are moments when cortisone, chiropractic, physical therapy, acupuncture, yoga, core strengthening and various forms of deep muscle therapy are all miraculous. But what do you do when all these treatments come up short? What do you do when surgery is thought to be the only remaining option? This is my point. When you fix enough of those cases, it teaches you something.

In the process of fixing chronic conditions variously diagnosed as a disc, arthritis, stenosis, spondylolisthesis, a bone spur etc., we get the entire purpose of orthopedic-neurological examination – to recreate the familiar pain the patient has been suffering. To hear the patient say, "That's it. That's my problem." You may not get that the first day, but definitely during the process, it's what we're looking for as we treat. This is what doctors look for in examination and tests like discography – yet do not find. This is a landmark in the history of spine medicine.

The source of pain so often attributed to joints and discs is actually cause by muscles, we just haven't been treating them correctly.

Summation

While we have the ability to visualize degenerated joints and discs on x-ray and MRI, we do not yet have the ability to see accurately the degenerated state of your muscles. And if we did, it would be the same as it is now for joints and discs:

- Healthy muscles and no pain, healthy muscles and lots of pain.

- Degenerated muscles and no pain, degenerated muscles and lots of pain.

It's not whether the joint or disc is symptomatic or not, it's whether your muscles are symptomatic or not. It's just that, so often, the symptoms feel nothing like a muscle.

It is the slightest injury to muscle fibers, or the aggravation of underlying spasm patterns that is the basis of back and body pain.

When your back goes out, what you have done is tweak muscle fibers in direct support of a weight bearing joint. In response to the tweak there is a reactive spasm in muscles around the injury. It is the reactive contraction crimping on joints that makes it feel deep in the joint. Radiating nerve pain down the leg is following a spasm pattern of muscle, it is not the sciatic nerve.

It is the reactive spasm from injury, crimping the disc that causes the inner jelly to squirt out like so much toothpaste out of the tube. As is so often observed, the body breaks down this extruded material, and discs routinely shrink or disappear on subsequent

DISC SHMISC

MRI, all on their own – yet symptoms remain.

Nerves exiting the spine are not as vulnerable as they appear. They are more like our own electrical chords that you could run over with a car yet not interfere with the current passing through them.

Back pain is self-limiting. For the masses, if you did nothing, it would go away on it's own. Your body makes a little bacon and you're right as rain. Many treatments work not because they recondition muscle, rather they help numb pain and spasm out of your awareness, which is what your body would do on its own. And this is why they don't work on tough cases — they do not recondition muscle, even if it is their stated goal. It is the reactive contraction from injury that never gets reconditioned properly and leads to chronic pain, and a feeling something isn't right.

What Griner figured out is — you can't beat muscles into submission, they will tense to resist. His genius take on stroking muscles one-time and releasing, finding a deck-of-cards feeling whether rolling flesh, crevice, or bone yields the entire purpose of orthopedic-neurological examination – the patient exclaiming, *That's it. That's my problem.* Finally, the source of chronic pain is revealed. The discrepancy in hard evidence makes sense, the disc is not the problem. Rather, an innocent bystander taking the blame for a crime it did not commit.

In my experience, fixing conditions variously diagnosed as a disc, arthritis, stenosis, a spondylo, a bone spur, etc., I'm not sure when these defects are ever the actual source of the problem.

Summation

So there you have it. Its been right in front of us all along, and as you can see, very understandable why we've been missing it. If you squeeze muscles like a piece of fruit, nothing sticks out. You can mash and steam roll muscles all day – it doesn't work on tough cases.

AMR – playing the body as a one-time deck of cards is the missing link to understanding back pain, and giving those who are suffering, the relief their body's been aching for.

The future

It is my contention that after a number of sessions, the patient comes to feel what it is we are working on and why. They know the different strokes involved in working their pattern, and to follow it's course becomes self-evident. If there was a machine that could reproduce the stroke, they could work on themselves. We need to take the money element out of it so people can put in the time it takes to achieve amazing results. The technology exists, investment is needed to design labor saving devices based on this technology. At the gym, where they have specific machines for pect, thigh and back, we'll have specific machines to recondition pect, thigh and back. Gyms will have sections devoted to self-therapy.

Or perhaps a new appliance, a robotic arm that no home can be without. Like the phone, the fridge, and the computer, how did we ever live without this?

When it comes to back pain, we'll look back on this period as the dark ages. What were we thinking? And what took so long to figure this out?

Hindsight is always 20/20

.

Appendix

Failure, Constitution, and Assorted cases

People will say, *Admit it, there must be some cases you couldn't fix, no?* Yes. Here's an assortment of cases that all have something to teach. There are a few chronic pain cases that didn't take a whole lot to fix, it just goes to show - you never know. In the last two cases, I discuss the principle of constitution.

Avascular necrosis of the hip

Marie taught ballet her whole life. Into her late 60's her body was as flexible and blithe as ever. She was the last person in the world she could imagine would have a problem with their body. The problem was her doctor had her on oral cortisone for a year, after complaining of stress and fatigue associated with her daughter being in a serious car accident.

DISC SHMISC

Several years later she noticed pain in the hip and groin that kept getting worse and worse until she couldn't walk on it. When I met her she was using a walker to get around. If you think of her body as a popsicle, her leg was the popsicle stick. Straight and stiff as a board, zero motion at the hip. You could try to pull her leg away from her body at the ankle and it would just twang in place.

The x-ray report is what bothered me most. While there was a decent looking hip and plenty of bone on x-ray, the report cited that because of her cortisone use she was predisposed to a condition called avascular necrosis.

Every bone has a tiny pinhole where a nutrient artery enters and feeds the living tissue of the bone. When the blood supply to the bone is cut off — avascular, necrosis — or cell death, sets in. The femur at the hip socket disintegrates.

I told her there was nothing I could do about avascular necrosis if that was the case, but I could tell her muscles were amazingly responsive for a woman her age.

In tough cases it is best to not look at a clock and work until you know you've given it a good "what for." It's different for everyone, for Marie it meant two-hour sessions. That was one tough leg. Often, it was "don't think, just work."

We did two-hour sessions three times a week for several months. We got all the motion back in the hip and leg, but she still couldn't put weight on it. I couldn't figure it out. An x-ray taken just a few months after we started showed that indeed she had avascular necrosis, the head of the femur had dissolved, there was nothing there to support her. She needed a hip replacement.

Her doctor told her the rule of thumb was: if you were able walk before surgery, it is likely you will be able to walk after surgery. But, if you were not able to walk before surgery, it is unlikely you would be able to walk afterward. Suffice it to say she recovered extremely well and had no trouble walking, she knows, in no small part to this work.

Years later she had the other hip replaced. I don't know whether she realized had it not been for the avascular necrosis she would not have needed a hip replacement. Also, surgery was covered by her insurance. Who can afford to pay out of their own pocket for the amount of treatment it may take to resolve their condition?

To this day, which is the "good" leg? The one we worked on.

Hypothesis: it is known that cortisone breaks down connective tissue. Add to that the reactive spasm of injury crimping concentrically around the deepest layers of muscle attaching to bone, and perhaps this is the mechanism of avascular necrosis?

Failure

There is only one case I regret. Just when you get a little cocky from fixing tough cases, life has a way of humbling you.

It was a personal injury case which I rarely do. I have what's called a cash practice. People normally pay me up front for services. Attorneys and insurance companies don't understand the necessity of long sessions, and the limited hours I can do this. In personal injury work, attorneys always expect your bills are "fluffy," and can be cut. I've fixed many tough cases doing regular hour sessions, and knowing we'd have some time, took it for granted it would break free as others had.

Dana was involved in an auto accident that left her with a deeply gripping right neck and shoulder pattern, along with other less serious injuries to other parts of the body. Shortly into treatment she was involved in another accident causing still more areas of complaint. When you're in pain, all areas that are screaming want some attention.

Appendix

While the minor areas went away, we never broke through the major neck and blade pattern, which was no different than Ted's case mentioned earlier, (page 118), and if anything, not quite as bad. I believe we were working too many areas in an hour session. I have no doubt we didn't break through the right neck and shoulder pattern because we didn't spend enough time there. What we did gave temporary relief, but not enough to break through.

Lesson learned? Never take results for granted. If you want to fix a tough case, you have to do what it takes.

Healing Power

At different times, Nina would implement different types of massage into her routine to take care of herself. About a year ago she had unusual symptoms she thought were stress related. It started with cramping and tingling in her shoulder, which is where she believed she carried her stress. It gradually became worse, then spreading into the neck, which became stiff and painful.

Months later it moved to the back of her head. Finally her eye was in a lot of pain. She thought it was a migraine, the back of the right eye would throb. Over-the-counter medications such as

Tylenol were of no help. She increased her massages feeling it was all connected to her shoulder.

"My eye was very dark on the top. My eye actually looked sunken in, it was like pulled back, which was very frightening. I thought ok, something is seriously wrong." She went to the eye doctor, who reported nothing wrong. She was now thinking it was a brain tumor and considering medical attention.

She also had a painful hard lump in the side of her chest wall near the breast, "It felt like cartilage". She saw a gynecologist who was puzzled by it. A mammogram and ultrasound could not determine what it was.

It happened that we were at a dinner and she was suffering miserably. I had her put her forehead in her hands on the dinner table, reached across the table and stroked the back of her head and neck for a few minutes while we waited for our meal. That five minutes gave her relief that lasted five days, while the one-hour massages she'd been getting gave her relief for 5 hours. This confirmed her suspicions that it had been coming from her neck, and knew she had to to give this work a try.

Appendix

After several months of weekly hour therapy the eye is clear, the lump is gone and she feels tremendous relief, "It's gone. It's gone. I think that was also related to this whole shoulder situation. I am much much better. I am extremely grateful. Because truly it works. It works. It's wonderful."

About four years ago she slipped and fell on an icy driveway in Chicago. "I landed on my hip and arm. I really believe that from that accident I did something to my shoulder. It never caused me any problems. It never caused me any pain. But it gradually and slowly got worse."

Lingering Effect Of Broken Leg

Susan broke her leg while traveling in a third world country. She literally hopped onto a plane, on one leg, to head for civilization and treatment.

The leg had to be re-broken, plates and screws inserted. She had a total of three surgeries on the leg and in the end the plates and screws were removed. While it never felt quite right, it healed up and she returned to running for exercise.

Over the years it became progressively worse until she was getting out of bed like a pirate with a peg leg. She tried acupuncture and massage but it kept getting worse.

She got some immediate relief of pain right from the start, not that it was fixed, it was a chronic problem that had developed over the course of years, and she understood it would take some doing.

At one point during the process, she started getting sharp nerve pain shooting through the heel upon planting her foot and pushing off to walk.

Despite the sharp pain, she knew overall she was getting better, and realized we were waking things up. After 7 months of weekly hour sessions we got a full resolution.

She said that ever since she'd broken the leg she'd never felt centered on that foot. She said she now felt centered again, and it's been holding steady.

This case points to the fact that we do not achieve our results by covering up pain. In the process of reconditioning chronic patterns we "wake things up," bringing fibers back online that were once plastered, and numbed out. Fortunately Susan understood the process.

Disc / Sciatica

Craig was diagnosed with a herniated disc causing radiating nerve pain down the leg, his calf and foot would go numb. When physical therapy, chiropractic, acupuncture, and injections of cortisone were unable to resolve his condition, surgery was recommended. Someone got him in to see me before that however.

Appendix

In this case it took a half dozen one-hour sessions to stabilize and life return to normal. What was it really? Nothing more than a spasm pattern from his butt down the leg. By working the pattern he came to feel the exact source of his pain.

Radiating Neck Pain

Sheila came in recently for a complaint in her low back, and reminded me of a condition we fixed fifteen years ago.

She had injured her neck and shoulder, causing a "buzzing", dull constant pain radiating all the way down her arm into the hand. It had been going on for four months and wasn't responding to chiropractic adjustments when she was referred in.

After 4-5 one-hour sessions she got up one day and the pain was gone. She kept waiting for it to come back, she had become so used to it. But it never came back.

"I felt the strength coming back and circulation coming back. When the pain was occurring, I could feel my deltoid atrophying. I could put my hand right there and I could just feel the bone. It was just flat. All the strength and power had gone away. It got healthy again. I felt great ever since then. It never came back."

DISC SHMISC
Flat feet

Mark had congenitally flat feet. When he changed careers and took a job that had him standing long hours, he was soon disabled with chronic foot pain. He'd seen several doctors, been given medication and tubing exercises, but months later he was still miserable. When he came in, his head was spinning with obsolete bits of information he'd picked up along the way. One treatment gave him relief like he'd never felt before. Four treatments later, he was stable.

Chronic Low Back Pain

Bob strained his lower back six years prior from lifting a heavy dryer. It got a little better, but had never really gone away. Over the years it deteriorated to the point where he was always wedging a towel or coat behind it for support when sitting in a car or at the movies, and bought a car with a lumbar adjustment.

Four one-hour sessions later, the pain went away and hasn't come back. That was over five years ago.

Chronic Wrist Pain

Years ago, Mel, Seth and I are driving to Palm Springs. It's July, and you could get golf packages really cheap.

Appendix

Mel announces that he won't be able to play due to wrist pain. It hurt to lift anything and made his job holding a camera for newspaper photography painful and difficult.

He had tried hitting a bucket of balls the night before and couldn't do it. He's just along for the ride as the package was non-refundable. I pull over to let Seth drive, and work on Mel's wrist the rest of the way.

He was then able to play, and we played 36 holes a day, two days in a row. Golfers will appreciate the kind of golfer Mel is: Seth and I are grabbing a sandwich between rounds, and Mel? He's out on the range hitting more balls. We play 72 holes of golf in two days and on the way back Mel announces his wrist is a little sore, and wants to let it rest.

Fast forward to next summer. I call Mel and suggest some golf. He says he can't play because of his wrist. I remind him the only reason he played last summer was because I worked on it.

When he comes to see me he admits that he saw an orthopedist last fall, "Because he's an orthopedist, you think he knows what he's talking about."

The doctor said that his wrist was no big deal and that a shot of cortisone would cure the condition. The relief was only temporary. The doctor suggested another but Mel refused.

Other recommendations were to wear splints for several months, which he also did not do. So he finally comes in, and 4 one-hour sessions later his wrist pain is gone. He plays golf regularly and it hasn't been a problem since. That was over ten years ago.

Conclusion: Who needs enemies? I have friends.

Constitution.

People have different constitutions, whether genetic, systemic or other, I don't know. I've had patients in their 60's, 70's and 80's with a healthy constitution. Their muscles aching to bust out and re-inflate with some proper reconditioning.

I've had patients in their 30's and 40's whose muscles were stubborn, and resistant to change.

Not so good constitution.

Mary, 40's, came in dragging her leg, radiating nerve pain to the foot, diagnosed with a 11mm disc herniation that, as usual, would later shrink to miniscule size on subsequent MRI. She'd tried physical therapy, chiropractic, acupuncture, and was now on the verge of disc surgery when she was referred in as a last resort.

She was no longer able to work, or participate in hobbies of sailing

144

and skiing, and had great difficulty just getting dressed in the morning. "I had to pick up my foot and deliberately place it in front of me in order to walk."

The muscles in her low back were as plastered as I've ever seen. She was giving me a chance, and it didn't feel like hour sessions were enough, so we went to hour and a half sessions twice a week. The term practice is just that, you practice and are not always sure of what you are doing.

Three months into treatment her husband returned from a ski trip one weekend to find his wife still miserable, and her leg all black and blue from me. He said, "Why are you messing around with this guy? Just get the surgery." I pleaded that we'd worked too hard to give up now.

It took four months until she experienced her first breath of fresh air, and feeling she could do things once again, promptly went out and planted a garden, which was a bit much and caused an exacerbation. Shortly after this, she was able to go snow skiing without incident.

To get at her low back we had to work up the leg, butt, and into her abdomen. In the process we recreated a waist and gave her a butt lift. At one point her friends thought she had lost weight when in fact she had gained ten pounds. We had changed the shape of her body.

DISC SHMISC

She got her life back: able to work, sailing and skiing, working on projects around the house, though never perfection.

The record is filled with being surprised how well it held up on vacation, or sitting at a 12-hour seminar, and also acute exacerbations from gardening, or sitting on a plane.

At different moments, the focus of pain, and thus the focus of treatment moved to the upper back, shoulder blade and arm. Other times it was headaches and neck pain.

We worked regularly over the course of a couple years. When we left off, she had occasional slight pain in the low back, occasional moderate pain in the low back associated with overdoing it, or sitting too long, and occasional slight pain in the leg.

(slight pain is pain you notice but doesn't hinder. moderate pain makes you alter how you do things.)

If you got that result from surgery, it would be deemed a great success. To me, it is what it is.

Mary had stubborn muscles, whether the cause is systemic, genetic or other, I don't know. They felt fibrotic and were resistant to change, though with massive treatment, obviously progress was made. While she had never been diagnosed with fibromyalgia, perhaps there is more than one form of the condition.

I learned a lot from working on her, and will admit to many mistakes. Many sessions there was so much I wanted to accomplish, no doubt at times I was too skippy, trying to cover too much ground, and not accomplishing much in any one.

While there are moments doing a little everywhere helps the system as a whole, sometimes you have to focus on an area and make a change.

We were doing hour-and-half sessions twice a week, and in her case I believe even longer sessions would have been valuable.

Good constitution.

Phyllis, 50's, comes in with chronic tightness in her neck and shoulders. Acupuncture, massage, stretching, and relaxation techniques were not getting it done. "Can I do half hour sessions twice a week?" Yes, you can do whatever you'd like. Did I have a clue this would suffice? No. In my mind I'm thinking it's chronic, she's in her 50's, it will never work.

Yet, she felt relief from day one, her muscles responded very nicely over the course of a couple months, she's thrilled, and we're not treating her anymore.

Her muscles had a very good constitution, they were aching to bust out and re-inflate with a little helping hand.

Thus, people's bodies have different constitutions. For some, a little AMR goes a long way. For others, it takes a lot to go a long way.

Made in the USA
Lexington, KY
26 February 2012